THE ULTIMATE GUIDE TO

the DANIEL FAST

THE ULTIMATE GUIDE TO

the DANIEL FAST

Kristen Feola

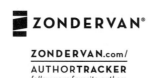

ZONDERVAN®

ZONDERVAN.com/
AUTHORTRACKER
follow your favorite authors

ZONDERVAN

The Ultimate Guide to the Daniel Fast
Copyright © 2010 by Kristen Feola

This title is also available as a Zondervan ebook. Visit www.zondervan.com/ebooks.

This title is also available in a Zondervan audio edition. Visit www.zondervan.fm.

Requests for information should be addressed to:

Zondervan, *Grand Rapids, Michigan 49530*

Library of Congress Cataloging-in-Publication Data

Feola, Kristen.
    The ultimate guide to the Daniel fast / Kristen Feola.
       p.   cm.
    Includes index.
    ISBN 978-0-310-33117-9 (softcover)
    1. Fasting—Religious aspects—Christianity. 2. Cooking—Religious aspects—Christianity. 3. Daniel (Biblical figure)
I. Title.
BV5055.F46 2010
248.4'7—dc22
                                           2010031941

Published in association with the literary agency of Les Stobbe, Literary Agent, lhstobbe123@gmail.com.

Cover design: Faceout Studio
Cover photography: Kristen Feola
Author photo: James Pauls, eyecrave photography
Interior photography: Kristen Feola
Interior design: Beth Shagene

Printed in the United States of America

10 11 12 13 14 15 /DCI/ 33 32 31 30 29 28 27 26 25 24 23 22 21 20 19 18 17 16 15 14 13 12 11 10 9 8 7 6 5 4 3 2 1

Contents

PART 3: The Food

Feast While You Fast

Blessed are those who hunger and thirst for righteousness, for they will be filled.
— Matthew 5:6

You're hungry, I can tell. You wouldn't be reading this book if you weren't. What you long for, though, isn't food. You're craving a different kind of nourishment.

Whatever you hunger for — direction for a job situation, healing from a devastating illness, wisdom in a relationship, freedom from an addiction, discernment for an important decision — know that the Lord will satisfy as you step out in faith and trust him to provide.

Although most people don't like the feeling of being famished, the Bible admonishes us to embrace it: "Like newborn babies, you must crave pure spiritual milk so that you will grow into a full experience of salvation. Cry out for this nourishment" (1 Peter 2:2 NLT). A baby's strongest desire is to have milk, and to have it as frequently as possible! It's only when we seek the Lord with this kind of determination that we can enjoy God's abundant provision of grace in our lives.

The Daniel Fast is a unique opportunity for you to hunger for the Lord and feast on the truth of his Word. When you fast, you restrict your food intake as a form of self-denial and worship, setting aside your basic physical desires for spiritual ones. You pull away from life's distractions and focus on your Savior so that you can be strengthened, refreshed, and renewed. God is ready to bless anyone who has an insatiable appetite for him and his Word. Those who long for the Lord and his righteousness will not be disappointed, because "he satisfies the thirsty and fills the hungry with good things" (Ps. 107:9).

So what do you say? Are you hungry for the Lord? Are you willing to empty yourself — of your needs, your plans, your dreams — so you can experience fullness in Christ? If so, then you're ready to begin the exciting twenty-one-day journey known as the Daniel Fast.

Why Fast?

Debra walked into work one day only to be informed by her principal that the teaching job she loved was coming to an end. It was a shock, to say the least. As a single mother supporting a

7

twelve-year-old daughter, she had no idea what she was going to do. However, Debra believed that the Lord had a plan, even though she couldn't yet see it. She decided to participate in the Daniel Fast to discern God's will for her life.

After only three years as husband and wife, Tyler and Hilary functioned more as roommates than as a young married couple in love. Financial problems and other issues had driven a huge wedge between them, causing distance in their relationship with each other and with God. Then Tyler recommitted his life to the Lord, and everything changed. Tyler and Hilary read the Bible together. They prayed together. They grew exponentially in the Lord. They entered into the Daniel Fast celebrating what God had done to restore their marriage and desiring to seek his direction for ministry. Both sensed that the Lord might be leading them to encourage other young couples with similar struggles. After seeing God transform their marriage in such a dramatic way, they were hungry for him to do more in their lives.

Michelle was sick and tired of being overweight. The year she turned forty, she sensed the Lord prompting her to do the Daniel Fast and to give him complete control over her eating habits. Michelle knew it was time to trust God to heal her from the emotional chains that had kept her bound in food addiction for years.

Maybe you're like Debra and could use divine wisdom to guide you. Perhaps you can relate to the problems Tyler and Hilary experienced, yet you've lost hope that anything will ever change. Or it could be that you know all too well what it's like to battle a life-controlling issue like Michelle has, and you are desperate for deliverance and healing. Whatever you are up against in your life right now, you are not alone. God sees your need. He wants you to cry out to him so he can come to your rescue.

Fasting is a powerful spiritual discipline that allows you to connect with God on a deeper level. When you fast, you deny yourself food, or certain foods, for a specified period of time as an act of surrender. You are, in essence, saying, "God, I have to have your help in this situation. I don't know what to do, and I'm willing to sacrifice my time, my physical comfort, and my desires so I can hear from you."

Fasting, when accompanied by fervent prayer, will help you develop intimacy with the Lord like nothing else can. Something supernatural happens when you humble yourself before God and pursue him with genuine passion. You experience a greater sense of his presence in your life, the indescribable joy that comes from walking in obedience, and God's richest blessings as you seek him wholeheartedly.

My First Daniel Fast

When I started my first Daniel Fast, I didn't know it would change my life. To give you a little background, a few years prior to the fast, I wrote a cookbook but never had it published. In fact, when I was in the final stages of editing it, the manuscript file somehow got corrupted, and I lost everything. One day I opened it up to make a few revisions, and the data was gone. The file was empty. I did have a hard copy of the cookbook, but it wasn't current, which meant I'd have to start over.

I set the cookbook aside for more than a year. Occasionally, I pulled out my notes and started working on it again, but I never felt the Lord's blessing when I did. Instead, I was anxious and stressed. I continued to sense that the Lord was asking me to wait, so I let the cookbook sit in a box on the top shelf of my closet.

Every so often, I glanced up at the box and heard a different voice: "You'll never finish. You're a failure." In those moments, I chose to listen instead to the voice of my Savior. Two particular verses sustained me during that time: "Wait for the Lord; be strong and take heart and wait for the Lord" (Ps. 27:14), and "I wait for the Lord, my soul waits, and in his word I put my hope" (Ps. 130:5).

Nearly two years after the incident with the cookbook, my church, James River Assembly, held a Daniel Fast in preparation for the launch of our second location, the Wilsons Creek Campus. We believed God was leading us to reach southwest Springfield, Missouri, with the love of Christ, but we needed his help. Our pastor, John Lindell, asked us to pray and seek the Lord's wisdom and favor as we stepped out in faith. A few days before Pastor John announced the churchwide fast, I had already planned to do a seven-day fast myself, and one of the main things I wanted to pray about was the cookbook. At that point, I was willing to do whatever God wanted, even if it meant the book would never be published. So when our pastor invited the congregation to join the leadership team by participating in a Daniel Fast, I felt excitement and anticipation. I knew God was about to do something amazing in my life and in the life of our church.

Early in the morning on day 1 of the Daniel Fast, I started a blog, thinking it would be fun to write about what I was experiencing and learning (*www.thosewhohunger.blogspot.com*). I never planned for the blog to be anything more than a journal. While cooking Marinated Zucchini that night for dinner, I thought, "This would be a great recipe for people doing the Daniel Fast." I mentioned it to my husband, and he suggested I post recipes on the blog for people in our church. The more I thought about the possibilities, the more excited I became. I began putting new recipes on the blog every day, many of them from my unpublished cookbook. As I did, God quietly whispered to my heart, "Do you see now? This is why I wanted you to wait. I had something bigger and better in mind."

That is how *The Ultimate Guide to the Daniel Fast* began. I'm still in awe that God took two things I love to do — cook and write — and combined them into one unbelievable blessing! The book you are holding is a testimony of the Lord's marvelous grace, which is best summed up by one of my favorite verses: "God can do anything, you know — far more than you could ever imagine or guess or request in your wildest dreams!" (Eph. 3:20 MSG).

How This Book Will Help You

Once you decide to do the Daniel Fast, it's important that you understand what your commitment involves. You certainly don't want to jump into your fast without first considering the time, attention, and energy you will need to invest in it.

Your first step is to formulate a plan. Without some kind of structure, you will more than likely struggle with frustration and discouragement. *The Ultimate Guide to the Daniel Fast* is your plan of action and your toolbox. It is divided into three parts:

PART 1: "The Fast"
PART 2: "The Focus"
PART 3: "The Food"

PART 1, "The Fast," explains what the Daniel Fast is, gives the biblical basis for the guidelines of the fast, explores fasting from God's perspective, looks at what fasting is and what it is not, and helps you create your fasting plan.

PART 2, "The Focus," delves into the spiritual component of your twenty-one-day adventure with the Lord, which is the reason you are fasting in the first place. You're sacrificing what you want physically because you're hungry for more of God. You have a desire to discern what he wants to accomplish in and through your life. This section of the book features twenty-one thought-provoking devotions that will strengthen your faith as you fix your eyes on Jesus. Each devotion also includes additional Scripture references to expand your study of the day's theme and a fasting testimony.

PART 3, "The Food," addresses the physical aspect of the Daniel Fast. It identifies the foods to eat and the foods to avoid, as well as provides more than one hundred tasty and nutritious recipes that are easy to prepare. This section also contains a suggested three-week meal plan, which will provide direction and show you how to organize the food component of your fast.

The journey on which you are about to embark is an exciting one. My prayer for you is that you will know the Lord more intimately as a result of your Daniel Fast experience and that you will be "filled to the measure of all the fullness of God" (Eph. 3:19).

Think of this book as a companion who will accompany you along the way. When you want ideas on what to cook for dinner, you can quickly and easily find a recipe. When you feel weary, you can be refreshed through Bible verses and devotions. When you are struggling with staying committed, you can refer to the information and tools in this book to motivate you.

Now that you have a better idea of how *The Ultimate Guide to the Daniel Fast* will help you, let's discuss what it means to participate in the Daniel Fast.

PART 1

the

FAST

So I turned to the Lord God and pleaded
with him in prayer and petition, in fasting.

—Daniel 9:3

Types of Fasts

When most people think of fasting, the first image that usually comes to mind is of a person going without food for several days and drinking only water, broth, and juice. Although fasting comes in a variety of forms, there are basically four types:

1. Absolute
2. Supernatural absolute
3. Liquid
4. Partial

An absolute fast is a fast from all food and liquids for a few days, which is what the apostle Paul experienced after the Lord appeared to him on the road to Damascus (Acts 9:9). Another example is when Queen Esther sent a message through Mordecai, asking the Jews to fast with her before she went to see the king. She said, "Do not eat or drink for three days" (Est. 4:16).

A supernatural absolute fast requires refraining from eating and drinking for a greater period of time than the absolute fast. It is referred to as supernatural because the length of time involved is medically impossible to survive without the divine empowerment of the Holy Spirit, such as when Moses went without food or water for forty days on Mount Sinai when he received the Ten Commandments from the Lord (Exod. 34:28).

A liquid fast involves eliminating food for a period of time and consuming only water, fruit juices, and vegetable juices. The Bible does not mention a liquid fast specifically, but it's an option that many people choose, especially when fasting for more than two or three days. This type of fast is not quite as taxing on the body as an absolute fast, and there is typically no danger of dehydration if adequate liquid is consumed.

On a partial fast, certain foods are removed from the diet for a specific length of time. The prophet Daniel chose to undergo a partial fast when he sought the Lord. His fasting experiences form the basis of the Daniel Fast.

The Daniel Fast

Participating in a Daniel Fast requires eliminating commonly enjoyed foods for twenty-one days as an act of worship and of consecrating oneself to God. Foods that are allowed are fruits, vegetables, whole grains, legumes, nuts, seeds, and oils. Restricted foods include dairy, meat, sugar, all forms of sweeteners, yeast, refined and processed foods, deep-fried foods, and solid fats. (For complete lists of foods to eat and foods to avoid, see p. 63.)

You don't have to be a spiritual giant to do a Daniel Fast. It's for anyone who is hungry for a deeper connection with the Lord and who is also willing to make a three-week commitment to the spiritual discipline of fasting as a means of pursuing that connection. Because it is a partial fast, as opposed to an absolute or liquid fast, participants are able to eat a wide variety of foods. For this reason, the Daniel Fast is a good entry-level fast. However, if you have a medical condition or any health concerns, you should consult with your physician before beginning any type of fast, including the Daniel Fast.

The guidelines of the modern-day Daniel Fast are based on the fasting experiences of the prophet Daniel. We follow his example not so much because his diet is worth emulating as because his heart is worth emulating. In the book of Daniel, chapters 1 and 10, we discover how Daniel's passion for God caused him to long for spiritual food more than physical food, which is the ultimate desire of anyone choosing to participate in a fast. As we take a closer look at what he did, it's important to remember that we're not trying to duplicate Daniel's menu, but we do want to imitate the spirit in which he fasted.

Daniel 1: The Ten-Day Test

The book of Daniel begins with a conquest. King Nebuchadnezzar of Babylon has besieged Jerusalem, the capital city of Judah, taken King Jehoiakim captive, and ransacked God's temple. As part of incorporating this new acquisition into his kingdom, Nebuchadnezzar brings a group of young Israelite men from their homeland to serve in his palace in Babylon — but not as prisoners or slaves. Nebuchadnezzar wants talent. He chooses the best — young men from wealthy, influential families, who are handsome, intelligent, and strong, with great poten-

tial for leadership and success. Nebuchadnezzar puts his chief official in charge of these men and commands that they be trained for three years before entering the king's service. Daniel is one of the king's young men, a captive Israelite brought to live in a pagan palace.

Each day the men receive a set amount of food and wine from the king's own table. However, Daniel resolves not to defile himself by partaking of the royal food. Most commentaries agree that the menu probably included food that had been sacrificed to idols and meat from unclean animals, such as pork, both of which were forbidden by Jewish dietary customs. Daniel wasn't being rebellious or obstinate by refusing to eat such food. He was simply unwilling to violate his convictions.

Daniel requests permission to eat only vegetables and to drink only water. The king's chief official is sympathetic but is afraid of the king's wrath if Daniel's limited diet causes him to look worse than the other men. Daniel then approaches the guard appointed to care for Daniel and three of his friends and proposes a test: "Please test your servants for ten days: Give us nothing but vegetables to eat and water to drink. Then compare our appearance with that of the young men who eat the royal food, and treat your servants in accordance with what you see" (Dan. 1:12 – 13). The guard agrees.

At the end of the ten-day test, Daniel and his friends look healthier and better nourished than the other young men who dined on royal food. From that point on, they are no longer forced to eat the king's food and have permission to eat only vegetables. The Bible says that to those four men who courageously stood up for their beliefs, God gave knowledge and understanding of all kinds of literature and learning. The Lord also gave to Daniel special insight and the ability to understand dreams and visions (v. 17).

What strikes me about this passage is that, despite the fact that Daniel was held captive by his enemies, he did not become a slave to fear. He knew that refusing the king's food might result in serious consequences, yet Daniel remained true to his convictions, demonstrating an unwavering trust in God. Although this particular experience wasn't technically a fast (since those foods most likely weren't part of Daniel's diet anyway), it's important to take a look at how he handled the situation so that we can better understand the man behind the fast mentioned in chapter 10.

I imagine too that the king spared no expense in what Daniel and the other men were served at mealtimes. The royal spread was probably unlike any food they had ever eaten — the best of the best. After all, Nebuchadnezzar was investing time and resources in training the men, and it was to his benefit that they be healthy and strong. Was Daniel tempted by the tasty food placed in front of him? Probably. The Bible doesn't say, so we can't know for sure. What we do know, however, is that if the king's food was a temptation for Daniel, he resisted it.

Just as Daniel faced trials in following the Lord, you undoubtedly will encounter challenges as well. The devil is outraged that you have committed to this fast, and he will find ways to place temptation in your path. To keep from being enticed into bondage by the enemy, you must prepare yourself for battle. As 1 Corinthians 16:13 advises, "Be on guard. Stand firm in the faith. Be courageous. Be strong" (NLT).

I want to encourage you to make time to be with the Lord over the next twenty-one days. I know, I know. You're busy. We all are. There are many people and things vying for your time, and sometimes it seems you can't fit them all in. Remember, though, that this is a fast, and fasting involves sacrifice.

Do all that you can to immerse yourself in the Word during your fast, and cling to God's promises. As you do, you won't become enslaved by anxiety, doubt, discouragement, or fear. You will walk in God's perfect peace, guarded by his truth. After all, it's the truth that sets you free, and if the Son has set you free, you are free indeed (John 8:36)!

Daniel 10: The Vision

Many years have passed since Daniel was a young man in King Nebuchadnezzar's palace. Daniel is now around eighty-five years old, and the Lord continues to reveal his purposes to him through dreams. In Daniel 10, Daniel receives a vision from God that disturbs him so greatly that he enters into a state of mourning, or fasting. God allows Daniel to foresee the many calamities that will befall the Jews for their sins, especially for destroying the Messiah and rejecting his gospel. Daniel is utterly distressed and sorrowful for his people and what they will have to endure.

The Bible says that he ate no choice food and had no meat or wine for three weeks (vv. 2 – 3). In the Hebrew text, the words translated "choice food," *chemdah* and *lechem*, indicate that Daniel refused himself foods that were desirable. Most commentaries agree that such desirable foods probably included bread and sweets. In the English Standard Version, Daniel 10:3 says, "I ate no delicacies," and another translation puts it this way: "I did not eat any tasty food" (NASB). Daniel ate simple foods, taking in only what was necessary for sustenance.

During his fast, Daniel was not focused on himself or his needs. He was broken and grieved in his spirit for the people he loved. We would do well to adopt this posture of prayer in crying out to God for our family and friends as we fast. Like Daniel, we have been given knowledge of what is in store for them if they continue to reject God's gift of salvation. That thought alone should cause us to fall on our faces before the Lord in fervent intercessory prayer.

A Biblical Perspective on Fasting

You won't find, "Thou shalt fast," anywhere in the Bible. However, there are a number of Scripture passages in both the Old and New Testaments that seem to imply that fasting will be a regular part of our lives.

Jehoshaphat declared a fast for all of Judah when he received word that their enemies were planning to attack them (2 Chron. 20:1 – 4). Ezra proclaimed a fast and prayed for a safe journey for the Israelites as they made the nine-hundred-mile trek to Jerusalem (Ezra 8:21 – 23). Nehemiah mourned, fasted, and prayed when he learned that Jerusalem's city walls had been broken down, leaving the Israelites vulnerable and disgraced (Neh. 1:1 – 4). Queen Esther asked all the Jews in Susa to fast and pray for her before she approached the king without an invitation from him, which could have resulted in her death (Est. 4:15 – 17). Anna, a prophetess, worshiped the Lord day and night in the temple, fasting and praying regularly (Luke 2:36 – 37). Finally, Jesus himself fasted for forty days and forty nights in the desert before beginning his public ministry (Matt. 4:1 – 11).

Perhaps one of the most descriptive passages about fasting, though, is found in Isaiah 58. In this chapter, the Lord is speaking to the Israelites through the prophet Isaiah, responding to the people's complaints about God's apparent indifference to their sacrifices: "'Why have we fasted,' they say, 'and you have not seen it? Why have we humbled ourselves, and you have not noticed?'" (v. 3).

Up to this point, the Israelites are doing everything by the book. They deny themselves food. They pray. And yet the Lord is not pleased. Where did they go wrong? What was the problem? The *Adam Clarke Commentary* suggests that God severely reproved the Israelites, calling their fasting hypocritical, because their behaviors in every other area of life were unjust and they exhibited no true repentance. In other words, they go through the motions of fasting but miss what it's all about. While they seem eager to know God and to follow his commands, they nevertheless continue to do as they please, exploit their workers, and quarrel among themselves to the point of getting into fistfights (vv. 2 – 4). God's response to their behavior is, "You cannot fast as you do today and expect your voice to be heard on high" (v. 4).

We should heed this warning if we want to fast and pray in a way that is acceptable to the Lord. The Israelites were fasting for all the wrong reasons. The mechanics of their fasting were right, but their hearts weren't, and it showed in how they lived their lives. To avoid repeating the mistakes of the Israelites, we need to ask the Lord to search our hearts and reveal any impure or selfish motives before entering into a fast. When he shows us, we must cry out to him in confession and repentance. Matthew Henry's Concise Commentary says of fasting, "A fast is a day to afflict the soul; if it does not express true sorrow for sin, and does not promote the putting away of sin, it is not a fast."[1]

Whole books have been written about the riches in Isaiah 58, but I want to summarize some key themes that have particular relevance not only for the Daniel Fast but also for understanding the foundation of a biblical perspective on fasting. If you haven't already, I encourage you to take a moment to read Isaiah 58 on your own. Read it slowly and prayerfully. Then, continue to review it over the next three weeks. As you consider the following themes, reflect on how you can apply them so that your Daniel Fast is a true fast in God's eyes.

Repentance

Acknowledging our sin to the Lord at the beginning of a fast is crucial. As we've seen in Isaiah 58, just because we fast and pray doesn't mean that God is pleased with our sacrifice. If our hearts are not right before him, any fasting we do will be meaningless and in vain. The Bible says, "Repent, then, and turn to God, so that your sins may be wiped out, that times of refreshing may come from the Lord" (Acts

3:19). When you are truly sorrowful over your sins, you lay the the foundation for God to restore you. The Lord will renew a right spirit in you, making you ready to undertake a fast that will be acceptable to him.

Sincerity

God is disgusted by hypocrisy in our lives. A hypocrite is someone who puts on a good front, pretending to be someone that he or she is not. When our lives reek of that type of deception, we really turn God off. The Bible says that when we cherish sin in our hearts, the Lord does not hear our prayers (Ps. 66:18). Such insincerity is why the Lord chastised the Israelites. On their days of fasting, they weren't focused on God. They were angry, argumentative, and violent. They were full of selfishness and guilty of manipulating others. Rather than submit to the Lord, they chased after their own desires. As a result, God rejected their fasting.

If you want your Daniel Fast to be pleasing to the Lord, begin by drawing near to him "with a sincere heart in full assurance of faith" (Heb. 10:22). Examine your motives for beginning this fast, and ask the Lord to purify you from any unrighteous attitudes or behaviors. When the Lord sees that your genuine desire is to honor him and to live a godly life, he will come near to you in return.

Intercession

Crying out to God for our own needs during a fast is important, but our prayers will be incomplete if we fail to intercede for others. Being

1. Matthew Henry, *Matthew Henry's Concise Commentary on the Whole Bible* (Nashville: Nelson, 2003), 688.

able to pray with and for people is an honor and a privilege. In my opinion, it's one of the greatest joys of fasting. It's also commanded by the Lord: "Confess your sins to each other and *pray for each other* so that you may be healed. The earnest prayer of a righteous person has great power and produces wonderful results" (James 5:16 NLT, emphasis added).

When the Lord challenges us in Isaiah 58:6 to "loose the chains of injustice and untie the cords of the yoke, to set the oppressed free and break every yoke," I believe he is calling us to cry out for those held captive by sin. According to the Forerunner Commentary, the purpose of fasting is "to free others from their sins, to intercede with God for their healing, to help provide for their needs, and to understand his will. Fasting is a tool of godly love we are to use for the good of others, and any benefits *we* derive from it are wonderful blessings!"[2]

Compassion

Fasting is both upward and inward. It's upward in the sense that your focus is on the Lord and his Word. It's inward because you are bringing your needs before the Lord in prayer, while simultaneously denying yourself certain foods as a sacrifice of worship to him.

Isaiah 58 shows us that fasting should also be outward, demonstrated through acts of compassion. Verse 7 describes how God wants us to reach out in his name: "Is it not to share your food with the hungry and to provide the poor wanderer with shelter — when you see

2. Richard T. Ritenbaugh, "Holy Days: Atonement," Forerunner Commentary, *www.bibletools.org*, "Bible Study," July 1996.

the naked, to clothe him, and not to turn away from your own flesh and blood?" This type of response is not one that expresses concern but does nothing when confronted with someone who has a need. It's a response of action. The resources that God has given us — money, possessions, talents, and time — are not bestowed upon us merely for our enjoyment. God intends for us to use them to bless others.

After camping out in this passage for a few weeks while writing this book, I realized that my fasts haven't even come close to what God requires. I was challenged by what I read and asked God to help me understand the verses in Isaiah 58 and how to apply them. For example, verse 10 says that for our fasts to be acceptable to God, we must "spend" ourselves "in behalf of the hungry." The phrase *spending ourselves* implies much more than just having good intentions. In the Hebrew, the meaning is "to draw out." To make this verse a reality in our lives, we can't sit on the sidelines. Instead, we must get involved and respond to the hurting people God places in our paths. By allowing the Lord to fill us with his compassion for others, we can help satisfy the needs of those he wants us to touch, both physically and spiritually. Reaching out to others might be as simple as writing a note of encouragement to a friend who is struggling, taking a bag of groceries to your local food pantry, cooking a meal for a family who has just lost a loved one or had a new baby, or giving someone you know a great big hug.

During your fast, prayerfully seek the Lord's direction as to how he wants you to spend yourself on behalf of those around you. Ask him to give you opportunities to bless others, and then get ready, because he will!

Reward

After studying God's requirements for fasting as outlined in Isaiah 58, you might feel the same way I do every time I read them — totally incapable of fulfilling such high standards. Don't despair! The Lord knows that we can't do it on our own. That's why he gave us the verse right in the middle of this passage that says, "Then you will call, and the LORD will answer; you will cry for help, and he will say: Here am I" (Isa. 58:9). I love the fact that he gave us that word of encouragement, knowing how overwhelmed we would feel! He also promises to guide us always, to satisfy our needs, and to strengthen us (v. 11), and he assures us that obedience in fasting results in blessing, healing, and protection. God says, "Your light will rise in the darkness, and your night will become like the noonday" (v. 10b), and, "You will be like a well-watered garden, like a spring whose waters never fail" (v. 11b). Finally, the Lord says we will find our joy in him. I can't think of a better reward!

What Fasting Is and What It Is Not

Fasting is mentioned repeatedly throughout Scripture, but unfortunately many Christians dismiss it as an Old Testament practice and unnecessary for today. Unwilling even to entertain the thought of denying themselves anything, they forfeit some of God's greatest blessings and miss out on knowing the Lord on a much deeper level.

Let's build on what we've learned about fasting up to this point with a few additional principles that will help expand our knowledge of this powerful spiritual discipline.

Fasting is the example set by Jesus.

First and foremost, we should fast because Jesus fasted. Before Jesus healed the ten lepers, before he raised Lazarus from the dead, and before he went to the cross, Jesus spent forty days and nights in the wilderness fasting and praying (Matt. 4:1 – 11). He didn't even begin his public ministry until he had spent that time alone with the Father in preparation for what God had called him to do. If Jesus, the Son of God, recognized the importance of fasting in his life, shouldn't we as well?

Fasting is an intense battle.

In Daniel 10, we get a glimpse of what occurs in the spiritual realm when we fast and pray. The Bible says that twenty-four days after he started his fast, Daniel was visited by a heavenly messenger, which most Bible scholars believe was the angel Gabriel. The angel said, "Do not be afraid, Daniel. Since the first day that you set your mind to gain understanding and to humble yourself before your God, your words were heard, and I have come in response to them. But the prince of the Persian kingdom resisted me twenty-one days" (vv. 12 – 13). Daniel's prayers were heard immediately, but the answers didn't come right away. There was a fierce battle in the heavenlies as Daniel prayed and fasted, and God's messenger was detained on the way by the opposition of the powers of darkness.

The battle is both physical and spiritual when you fast. First, you are at war with your own flesh — your body and its passions — because your flesh wants no part of it. Also, you're fighting against the enemy of your soul, whose ultimate goal is to defeat you. But you don't need to be paralyzed by fear. The all-powerful, all-knowing, almighty God is on your side. He fights for you and will give you victory as you trust in him. Remember, you are more than a conqueror in Christ (Rom. 8:37). The battle has already been won!

Fasting gives us victory over the enemy.

After fasting forty days and forty nights in the desert, Jesus was hungry. When Satan appeared and offered him some bread, Jesus must have been tempted to take it. After all, he hadn't eaten anything for more than a month. Instead of giving in, though, Jesus resisted the enemy's attack by speaking truth. Matthew 4:4 says, "Jesus told him, 'No! The Scriptures say, "People do not live by bread alone, but by every word that comes from the mouth of God"'"(NLT). Satan was persistent, though, and tempted Jesus two more times from two different angles. In both cases, Jesus responded to his attacks with the Word of God.

Jesus' example makes it quite clear what we need to do to walk in victory. We must equip ourselves for battle by fighting with the sword of the Spirit (Eph. 6:17). The Word is our weapon of warfare, and this weapon has divine power (2 Cor. 10:4). As you meditate on truth and let it sink deep within you, the Holy Spirit will give you strength to stand firm and not fall. When you study God's Word, you'll be able to recall applicable verses during times of tempta-

tion. The Holy Spirit will bring those memorized verses to your mind, and you will have victory not only during this twenty-one-day period of fasting but also in the weeks, months, and years that follow.

Fasting empowers us for ministry.

When members of the church at Antioch were worshiping the Lord and fasting, the Holy Spirit instructed them, "Set apart for me Barnabas and Saul for the work to which I have called them" (Acts 13:2). The Bible says that after they had fasted and prayed, the members of the church laid hands on Paul and Barnabas and sent them off. This example shows us that one of the benefits of fasting is that it anoints us with power for what God has planned for us to do.

Fasting acknowledges our complete dependence on God.

The Bible says that God has set eternity in our hearts (Eccl. 3:11), which means he has created within each of us a void that only he can fill. Therefore, it is literally in our DNA to long for God. However, we can easily be deceived and believe the lie that we don't really need God and that we can make it on our own. Pride and self-sufficiency crowd out any desire for the Lord, and soon our hearts become hardened to his working in our lives.

Fasting provides a much-needed shock to our systems and jolts us back into a right way of thinking. We're humbled as we realize how completely dependent we are upon the Lord and his mercy. The physical weakness we experience helps us to remember that the Lord is the one who sustains us and that only he truly satisfies.

Fasting is about food.

In every instance of fasting in the Bible, people either go without food or a combination of water and food. A popular Christian practice in our culture today is to declare a fast from other things, such as shopping, using a computer, or watching television. Although these self-denials have benefits, they are not fasts according to biblical examples.

Abstaining from food or groups of foods, such as on a Daniel Fast, results in a deep spiritual awareness that doesn't come by fasting from the mall or your favorite sitcom. You don't experience uncomfortable hunger pangs when you decide to take a break from the internet for a week. However, when you eliminate food that you like and eat regularly, your body will make you miserable until you give it what it wants. For example, if you normally drink coffee first thing in the morning, your body will communicate its desire for caffeine by blessing you with a severe headache!

The physical side effects and cravings that you endure while fasting serve as constant reminders that you desperately need the Lord every minute of every day. You understand this dependence in a greater way when food restrictions are involved, because the struggle is both spiritual and physical. That is why for a fast to truly be a fast, it must involve self-denial of food.

Fasting is not about food.

While self-denial of food is a necessary component of the Daniel Fast, you must not let it take center stage. As difficult as it may be, especially at the beginning of the fast, resist the temptation to get so caught up in what you're going to eat that you lose sight of the many benefits of fasting: physical and spiritual cleansing, heightened spiritual sensitivity, joy in serving others, and sweet fellowship with the Lord. If you become consumed with food and fail to seek the Lord, then all you're doing is a twenty-one-day diet.

Fasting is about you.

Jesus said, "Come to me, all of you who are weary and carry heavy burdens, and I will give you rest" (Matt. 11:28 NLT). The Lord *wants* you to bring your needs before him. Consider the Daniel Fast to be a personal invitation from your Father God. He is giving you a unique opportunity to draw closer to him. Psalm 103:11 says, "For as high as the heavens are above the earth, so great is his steadfast love toward those who fear him" (ESV). The Lord loves you and cares about every detail of your life. If something matters to you, then it matters to him. In this sense, fasting *is* all about you. Whatever you need to receive from the Lord during your fast — whether it's encouragement, discernment, healing, hope, strength, or wisdom — know that the Lord desires to give it to you. He longs to give such good gifts to his children (Matt. 7:11). He's just waiting for us to ask.

Fasting is not about you.

Your fast is not at all about you or what you want. It's about God and what *he* wants.

In Zechariah 7, the Israelites ask the priests whether they should fast as they had in the past. The Lord speaks to the prophet Isaiah, saying, "Ask all the people of the land and the priests, 'When you fasted and mourned in the fifth and seventh months for the past seventy years, *was it really for me that you fasted?'"* (Zech. 7:5, emphasis added).

Ouch. That's a piercing question not only for the Israelites but also for us. It challenges us to examine our motivations for undertaking a fast. Do we truly want to fast as an act of obedience and worship? Or are we trying to manipulate God and twist his arm to answer our prayers the way we want him to? It's important to discern our true intentions and then to surrender them all to God. A fast that honors God requires that we release the stranglehold we have on our lives and submit to the Lord. We worship and praise him not for what he can give us but for who he is. We give all of ourselves in loving obedience and service because we believe wholeheartedly that the best place we could ever be is in the center of God's will.

Fasting is life-changing.

Fasting is an act of humility that is rewarded by the Lord. He is pleased when we make God-honoring sacrifices in order to draw close to him. Here's a promise you can count on: "Come near to God and he will come near to you" (James 4:8). The Bible also says that God blesses us when we seek him: "Humble yourselves before the Lord, and he will lift you up" (James 4:10).

Whenever we spend time in the Lord's presence, we are changed. His Word transforms us and renews our minds, making us more sensitive to the Holy Spirit's activity in our lives. By reading God's Word and meditating on it, we will think truth, speak truth, and act out the truth. The more time we spend in the Word, the more we will look like Jesus. Talk about life-changing!

After reading this far, you may be feeling a little overwhelmed. Perhaps you're considering all the different components of fasting, wondering if you can do it. Let me assure you that you *can* do it, because the Lord will empower you to fulfill your commitment. He is faithful and will walk with you every step of the way.

Fasting is a magnificent multifaceted mystery. It's impossible for us to grasp the scope of it with our finite minds. However, fasting is more than physical self-denial. When coupled with fervent prayer, fasting opens the way for God to step in and do miraculous things in our lives and in the lives of the people around us.

I hope that after reading the information in this section, you see fasting as an exciting adventure and not a long list of rules. The last thing I want for you to do is throw your hands up in frustration and let out a big sigh, thinking, "Wow. I had no idea fasting is that complicated!" Fasting, in essence, is really quite simple. Focus your energy on the following five things and you will have done your part to experience a successful Daniel Fast. The rest will be up to God.

1. Pray often.
2. Read the Word daily.
3. Believe God's promises.
4. Restrict your food intake.
5. Praise and thank the Lord!

Now let's examine how creating a fasting plan can help you stay organized and ensure that your fast is as effective as possible.

Creating Your Fasting Plan

Before the Fast

A week before your fast, prepare spiritually and physically for what you are about to undertake. My advice is that you go through the following list and complete as many of the tips as you can. Don't worry if you aren't able to implement everything. The Lord will bless your efforts to get ready for your fasting experience.

Spiritual Preparation

1. *Identify your primary motivation for fasting.* Ask yourself why you are doing the Daniel Fast. Do you need wisdom in making a decision? Do you desire physical healing? Do you want to intercede for a family member or a friend who doesn't know the Lord? Once you have answered that question, pray and thank God for his provision. Trust that he will answer as you seek him. Also, think about other prayer requests you have for yourself and others, and make a list of those needs.

2. *Decide on a Bible reading plan.* The daily devotions in this book are intended to be a springboard that launches you into the Word. One way you can supplement the devotional material is to look up the additional Scripture references that are given each day. The verses will help to draw you into deeper study of the devotion's main theme. Another option for a simple study plan during your fast is to choose a book of the Bible and read several verses out of it each day. Something that has also worked well for me is to read the psalm and proverb that correspond to the date on the calendar. For example, on January 1, my daily reading would be Psalm 1 and Proverbs 1. Whatever you decide to do, make sure you find a system that is reasonable and fits the length of time you will spend in the Word each day.

3. *Read Isaiah 58 and other verses on fasting.* Studying such passages will help you to align your heart and mind with what God desires for a fast. Reread the section "A Biblical Perspective on Fasting" (p. 16) and revisit the verses mentioned in the section "What Fasting Is and What It Is Not" (p. 19) for additional insight.

4. *Ask a friend to be your prayer partner.* Having someone pray with you and for you throughout your fast is a wonderful benefit and a source of encouragement. Ideally, your prayer partner should be someone who is also doing the Daniel Fast, but that is certainly not a requirement. The key is that you have someone who will lift your needs up in prayer and keep you accountable.

5. *Buy a journal or use a notebook.* God is going to do many amazing things during your fast, and it's a good idea to write them down. Use a journal for prayer requests, praises, and answers to prayer, and to record what the Lord shows you through his Word.

Physical Preparation

1. *Ease into the fast.* The week before your fast begins, start cutting back on the amount of meat, dairy products, caffeine, and sugar you consume. Doing so will help your body slowly adjust to the Daniel Fast food guidelines and should also reduce the severity of any unpleasant side effects that might occur. Also, increase your water consumption, as well as your fruit and vegetable intake.

2. *Plan your meals for the first week.* The key to success with the food portion of the fast is proper planning. It will end up saving you time in the long run, help prevent the frustration of trying to decide at the last minute what to eat, and keep you from indulging in foods that don't fall within the guidelines of the fast. Take advantage of the fact that some of the meal planning for your fast has already been done for you! On pages 65 – 67 are suggested meal plans for each week. These meal plans are helpful in that they limit the number of recipes you choose from, making it a little easier to get a handle on creating your meal plan, yet still give you the freedom to tailor the meal plans according to your tastes and needs. Refer to "Creating Your Daniel Fast Meal Plan" on page 64. You can also find substitutions for any of the suggested recipes by using the index (p. 219) to locate alternative recipes that you might like to try.

3. *Make a grocery list for the first week.* If you are using the suggested meal plans, appendix 3, the "Daniel Fast Menu Planning Tool" (p. 203), will make putting together your grocery shopping lists a little easier.

4. *Prepare food ahead of time.* Look at the first week's recipes to find ways you can speed up food preparation and make it more efficient. For example, if Tuesday's lunch recipe calls for cooked brown rice, make the rice Monday night or Tuesday morning. Another way to save time is to cut up the fresh vegetables that are called for in that week's recipes and store them in the refrigerator until you're ready to use them.

5. *Cook and freeze meals.* Carve out a few hours the weekend before your fast kicks off to make three or four of the recipes for week 1, such as Black Bean Chili Bake, Hummus, and Tuscan Soup. You can also store half of what you make in airtight containers in the freezer for later in the fast. (Be sure to label them.)

During the Fast

Focus on the Lord, and make him your top priority over the next three weeks. You may feel tempted to cheat, compromise, or even quit along the way, but don't. God will give you the self-control and perseverance you need to complete your fast. Be strong in the Lord and in his mighty power!

Spiritual Preparation

1. *Get alone with God every day.* Read his Word and pray. This is a must. You cannot neglect time with the Lord and expect your fast to be effective.

2. *Go through the devotions in part 2, "The Focus" (p. 33).* Read each day's entry and meditate on what God shows you through his Word.

3. *Review appendix 2, "Verses to Feed On" (p. 201).* Continually refer to these precious nuggets of truth, especially when you need encouragement. Be sure to say the words aloud as well. Speaking the Word instead of merely reading it gives you strength and builds your confidence in the Lord.

4. *Be in contact with your prayer partner to share how he or she can continue to pray for you.* Celebrate ways in which God has provided and how he has answered prayer.

5. *Write down what God reveals to you.* Record insights that the Lord gives you, along with prayer requests and praises.

Physical Preparation

1. *Drink plenty of water.* Daniel Fast foods are rich in fiber, so it's essential that you provide your body with the water it needs for the amount of fiber you're consuming. Drink water throughout the day. Carry a water bottle around with you, or have a large cup of water on your desk at work. Don't wait until you're thirsty to drink, either. If you wait until you feel the thirst sensation, you're probably already slightly dehydrated. Insufficient water intake is also a primary cause of constipation, which you definitely want to avoid on your fast. Your daily goal is to drink about half your body weight in ounces of water. For example, someone who weighs 150 pounds should be consuming approximately seventy-five ounces of water, or about nine cups, each day. That may sound impossible, but remember that you are ingesting a significant amount of water through the food you're eating, which counts toward your goal. The table on this page gives you an idea of what you need to drink. I hope you don't feel water-logged just by looking at it! The best way to increase your water consumption during your fast is to do it gradually. If you usually drink around two cups of water per day, try to drink two to three cups and work your way up to more. One way to determine if you're drinking enough water is to check the color of your urine. It should be almost colorless to light yellow. If the color is dark, you're probably dehydrated.

Body Weight (pounds)	Daily Water Consumption Goal (cups)
100 – 125	6 – 8
125 – 150	8 – 9
150 – 175	9 – 11
175 – 200	11 – 12
200 – 225	12 – 14
225 – 250	14 – 16
250 – 300	16 – 18
300 – 325	18 – 20
325 – 350	20 – 22

2. *Plan your meals for weeks two and three.*

3. *Continue to refer to the meal plans for each week for ideas.*

4. *Make a grocery list for weeks two and three.*

5. *Prepare foods ahead of time.*

6. *Double recipes and freeze them.*

7. *Improve digestion by eating slowly and chewing your food well.* Our lives are fast-paced, and this tendency to be in a constant rush often carries into our eating habits. Instead of enjoying our food,

we inhale it, which often results in bloating, indigestion, and over-eating. Slow down at mealtimes. Don't be in such a hurry. Savor the good food God has given you. Your body will thank you for it.

8. *Try juicing.* Juicing used to be one of those activities that only weird, way-out-there people did. Now, more and more people are realizing the benefits of fresh fruit and vegetable juices. If you've never tried juicing, you should consider adding a juicer to your birthday or Christmas list. Juicing is really ideal for a Daniel Fast because you are able to take in a variety of fruits or vegetables at one time. Another selling point for juicing is that it's a big hit with kids! My daughters love to help me make fresh juice. Getting kids involved in making the juice more than likely increases the chances of their actually drinking it. (A word of advice, though, is to start with something you know they will like, such as apple juice, grape juice, or orange juice. Don't try anything fancy at first. Later you can sneak in other foods: broccoli, carrots, celery, etc.) Refer to the section "Juices" (p. 188) for recipe ideas. A few of the benefits of juicing are:

   • Fresh juices are easily assimilated, absorbed, and digested.
   • Juicing allows you to consume a variety of fruits and vegetables in an efficient manner.
   • Your body receives an instant boost of nutrients, enzymes, vitamins, and minerals in a form that it can use quickly.

9. *Focus on foods you can eat, not on foods you can't eat.* All of us can think of a food item that we will miss while on the Daniel Fast. For me, it's green tea with honey. Others will count the days until they can have their favorite soft drink or coffee. Most men can't wait to have a thick, juicy hamburger or steak once the fast is over. While we're fasting, we shouldn't complain or be grouchy because we're not able to enjoy what we're used to having (Phil. 2:14). Fasting is a time of self-denial; it's not supposed to be comfortable. Remember that your Daniel Fast is a voluntary act of worship. You have chosen to do it. Maintain an attitude of gratitude by continually thanking the Lord for the food you are eating, just as the Bible says to do in 1 Thessalonians 5:18: "Give thanks in all circumstances, for this is God's will for you in Christ Jesus."

10. *Exercise.* Perhaps exercise is already a part of your life and you reap the benefits of it each week. Maybe, though, the e-word is like an infectious disease, and you avoid it at all costs. Whatever your activity level, consider that the Lord commands us to honor him with our bodies (1 Cor. 6:19–20). I believe exercise is one way he expects us to care for ourselves. If you are not already working out regularly, now just might be the time for you to begin a basic exercise program. It can be as simple as going for a walk or riding your bike two to three times a week. Once you allow God to transform your thinking in this area so that you see exercise as a privilege rather than a punishment, you will experience the joy of knowing that you are caring for your body in a way that is honoring to him.

After the Fast

Congratulations! You have successfully reached the end of your journey, and now your Daniel Fast is complete. Way to go! I hope you feel so energized that you are determined to continue eating this way. However, I realize that you might be ready to say goodbye to beans, vegetables, and rice for a while so you can enjoy your favorite foods once again. Following are a few guidelines to help you as you break your fast.

Spiritual Preparation

1. *Continue to spend time in the Word each day.*

2. *Continue to pray.*

3. *Continue to journal.*

Physical Preparation

1. *Ease out of the fast.* After depriving yourself of your favorite foods for three weeks, you may experience strong cravings for them. In fact, you may even have planned on day 1 of the fast exactly how you would break the fast as soon as it was completed! Resist the temptation to go overboard. For your first post-fast meal, don't make the mistake of stuffing yourself at your favorite restaurant. You'll regret it if you do! Give your body time to adjust to foods you

haven't eaten in twenty-one days. Take it slow and limit yourself to small portions. It might be helpful to plan your meals for the first couple of days after your fast is completed to avoid overeating.

2. *Continue to drink water.* For the past three weeks you have consumed gallons of water, and it would be a shame for you to let this positive new habit fall by the wayside. The following list identifies a few of the many reasons why our bodies need water to survive and thrive. Some of the functions of water are:
   - Enables the body to metabolize stored fat.
   - Helps to maintain proper muscle tone.
   - Lubricates joints.
   - Prevents and relieves constipation.
   - Prevents heartburn.
   - Reduces fluid retention.
   - Regulates body temperature.
   - Rids the body of waste.
   - Suppresses the appetite naturally.

3. *Continue to make healthy choices.* Throughout your fast, you relied on the Lord's strength to abstain from certain foods as an act of worship to him. You put God first and did your best to make healthy choices. Even though your fast is over, it's still important that you take care of your body. If the fast revealed any food addictions you have, be aware of those temptations as you resume "regular" eating. Just as one drink can send an alcoholic into a downward spiral, so can a single bite of a sugary food trigger an eating binge for some people. Sugar can be just as addictive as drugs or alcohol. Rather than giving in to our cravings, we need to ask the Lord for wisdom to avoid foods that are problematic for us. He will help us overcome temptation so that we can walk in victory and live "self-controlled, upright and godly lives" (Titus 2:12). Remember what the Lord has shown you throughout your fast, and do not return to destructive eating habits that could hinder your spiritual growth. Make an effort to choose foods that provide the nourishment your body needs. In addition, if you began an exercise program during your fast, continue to make regular physical activity a part of your life. If you haven't yet tackled that goal, make plans to do it.

PART 2

the

FOCUS

I have chosen the way of truth;
I have set my heart on your laws.

—Psalm 119:30

Focus on God by Feasting on His Word

When your words came, I ate them; they were my joy and my heart's delight,
for I bear your name, O LORD God Almighty.

—Jeremiah 15:16

One of the most spectacular events that occurs in nature is the metamorphosis of a caterpillar into a butterfly.

A lowly, ground-crawling caterpillar is miraculously changed into a brightly colored winged creature that soars high in the sky. It's a beautiful illustration of what needs to happen in our lives if we are to be transformed into the image of Christ.

Caterpillars have one goal — to eat. Every day, they consume as much food as possible. Eating is the focus of their existence, which causes them to grow very quickly. In their short lifetimes, caterpillars consume as much as twenty times their weight. The caterpillar must take in this much food to prepare for the next stage of its development, which is to form the chrysalis. Inside the chrysalis, new body parts are formed. This process takes weeks, and sometimes even months. When the time is right and the changes are complete, a magnificent butterfly breaks through its shell and emerges, looking nothing like the caterpillar it once was.

For the next twenty-one days, you need to occupy yourself with the spiritual equivalent of caterpillar consumption. Spending time in God's Word is vital to the success of your fast. Devour as much as you can. Make reading the Bible your top priority, and stuff yourself full of God's truth. Eat and eat and eat and eat. If you do, you won't stay the same. Your thoughts, attitudes, and actions will change. You will grow in Christ and "be transformed by the renewing of your mind" (Rom. 12:2). As you submit to the Lord and savor every morsel of his powerful Word, he will shape you into who he has created you to be. You won't look like the old you any longer. Instead, you will begin to look more like Jesus.

In this section, you will find twenty-one daily devotions, each of which features additional Scripture references for further study, along with a fasting testimony. The devotions are divided into the following themes:

WEEK 1: Repentance and Praise
WEEK 2: Trials and Perseverance
WEEK 3: Trust and Transformation

Focus on the Lord, feast on his Word, and, like the butterfly, you will soon witness a metamorphosis in your life. Open up your heart to him, start stretching your wings, and get ready to fly.

Fasting Begins with Confession

*If we confess our sins, he is faithful and just and will
forgive us our sins and purify us from all unrighteousness.*
— 1 John 1:9

Today is an exciting day as you set out on your Daniel Fast journey. God has much to show you, so it's important that you get started on the right foot. Since the purpose of fasting is to seek God through prayer, it only seems right that on day 1 we look at how Daniel approached the Lord.

One day, when Daniel was studying the words of Jeremiah the prophet, he was greatly troubled by what he read. He understood from the Scriptures that the Israelites were going to suffer for many years to atone for their rebellion against the Lord. Daniel's immediate response was to fast and pray. His words are recorded in Daniel 9 and lay the foundation for how we should begin this Daniel Fast.

Daniel's first words acknowledged his sin and the sin of his people. In verses 4 – 10, we see phrases such as "we have sinned and done wrong," "we have been wicked," "we have turned away from your commands," "we have not listened," and "we have not obeyed." Daniel knew it was necessary for the Lord to purify him from the unrighteous behaviors in his life before his time of prayer and fasting could be effective.

Why start with confession? Our God is a holy God, and when we live in willful disobedience, our sins prevent us from enjoying sweet fellowship with him. Confession breaks down the barriers that stand in the way of his full blessing in our lives.

As you spend time in prayer today, ask God to reveal your attitudes and behaviors that do not line up with his Word. As he brings those sins to your mind, confess them. Agree with the Lord that you have been wrong. Once that has been done, receive his forgiveness and mercy. Then, thank him for cleansing you and purifying you from all unrighteousness.

You are now ready to move forward. God has led you to do this Daniel Fast, and he has much to do in and through your life over the next three weeks. Expect great things, because our God is a great God!

> You have to do a Daniel Fast for the right reasons. I entered into the fast because everyone around me was doing it and because I thought it would help me lose weight. At no point did I increase my prayer time or treat it as anything more than a diet program. So it's no surprise that I made it only halfway through the fast, and I didn't get any closer to God in the process. I felt like a failure. The next time I do a Daniel Fast, I will make sure that I partner with God. It will be less about me and more about him.
> — K. MOORE

***Verses for
additional study:***
Psalm 38:18
Psalm 51:2
Proverbs 28:13

Lord, show me any areas in my life that are not pleasing to you. I turn away from my sins and turn to you, O God, so that I can begin this fast with a clean conscience and a pure heart. I'm excited about what you are going to do over the next three weeks!

Go to Mount Moriah

You shall have no other gods before me.

—*Exodus 20:3*

I'm being stalked by a guy named Abraham. He follows me everywhere — my Bible study lesson, the Wednesday-night prayer service, the book I'm reading. What is it with this guy, and what does he want with me? Okay, maybe I'm a little slow, but I'm starting to think God is trying to get my attention, and he is using the story of Abraham to do it.

Perhaps you're familiar with the account. God promised Abraham that he would be the father of many nations. However, at age ninety-nine, Abraham and his wife, Sarah, were still waiting for a baby. When he turned one hundred, though, the most incredible thing happened. They had a son! Abraham's greatest longing was fulfilled, and Isaac was his joy.

Years later, God told Abraham to take his beloved Isaac to a mountain to sacrifice him as a burnt offering. Why would God ask Abraham to do such a horrific thing? The Lord was testing Abraham to see whether the love he had for his son was greater than the love he had for his Lord. Although Abraham's heart was broken at the thought of harming Isaac, he got up early the next morning to set out for Mount Moriah. Abraham knew that to obey God, he had to place Isaac on the altar.

Just as Abraham raised the knife to take his son's life, an angel of the Lord spoke to him and told him not to lay a hand on the boy. God provided a ram caught in a nearby thicket to be the burnt offering instead.

It wasn't wrong for Abraham to love Isaac. The problem was that Abraham loved him a little too much. In the book *Counterfeit Gods*, author Timothy Keller makes this observation: "If God had not intervened, Abraham would have certainly come to love his son more than anything in the world, if he did not already do so. That would have been idolatry, and all idolatry is destructive."[3]

Verses for additional study:

Genesis 22:1 – 18
Exodus 20:4
Psalm 24:3 – 5
Isaiah 42:8

3. Timothy Keller, *Counterfeit Gods: The Empty Promises of Money, Sex, and Power, and the Only Hope That Matters* (New York: Dutton, 2009), 13.

Are there any idols in your life? God calls us all to surrender our "Isaacs" to him. Don't be afraid to climb Mount Moriah. Go now, and don't hesitate. Lay it all on the altar. Your Provider will meet you there and deliver you, just as he delivered Abraham.

Dear God, show me if I have any "Isaacs" in my life. Give me the strength and courage to dethrone things that I have placed before you. You are my Master. I serve you and you alone.

The Daniel Fast is my fast of choice when I need direction or refreshment, or desire to hear God's voice more clearly. This daily, living sacrifice is a wonderful way to establish a constant awareness that I am reprioritizing my life, putting all idols away, and allowing God to reign in my heart. God has shown me time and time again that when we bring our appetites and flesh under the direction of his Spirit, he will reward. I am always touched by how God honors our efforts, no matter how small. Not because we have to work for his approval but because he is so full of grace and looks for opportunities to bless us. Fasting is one of those gracious opportunities.

— S. HORD

DAY 3

His Glorious Name

Praise be to his glorious name forever;
may the whole earth be filled with his glory.
— Psalm 72:19

When I was pregnant, I spent hours flipping through books of baby names trying to find just the right name for our little one. We finally decided on Isabelle for our firstborn, which means "consecrated to God," and Jocelyn for our second daughter, which translates "joyful spirit." It was important to us that our children have names that not only sound nice but also are rich in meaning.

The Bible gives several examples of how people's names often describe their character or behavior. For example, during the first part of his life, Jacob lived up to his name of "trickster" by deceiving his brother, Esau, and his father in order to obtain Esau's birthright. Later in Jacob's life, after he wrestled with the Lord and finally submitted to him, God changed his name to Israel, meaning "straightened by God."

When you choose to follow the Lord and receive his gift of salvation, you're also given a new name. You become a Christian, which means "follower of Christ." However, you don't earn the right to bear his name

Verses for additional study:
Genesis 25:29 – 34
Genesis 27:1 – 40
Genesis 32:22 – 28
Genesis 35:10
Psalm 113:2 – 3
Ephesians 2:8 – 9
Titus 3:5

because of your righteousness. Your good works don't give you the privilege of identifying with the Lord. No, the only reason you carry his glorious name is because of Jesus and what he did for you.

Jesus paid a high price to call you his own. He loved you so much that he was willing to die to give you life. Spend a few moments now thanking God for sending Jesus so that you could be set free from sin. Praise the Lord for his infinite mercy and love!

Father God, I praise you! My mind cannot fathom the depths of your love. Thank you for sending Jesus for me so I could be a part of your family and live with you for eternity.

Our family participated in a Daniel Fast with our church last year. The first couple of days, I really struggled with the food and what I was giving up. I had horrible headaches and thought that twenty-one days felt like an eternity. Yet as I began to focus on the purpose of the fast, I felt like God offered me a handwritten invitation to "go deeper" with him. Accepting that invitation helped me to experience a level of intimacy and a tender worship I never knew before participating in the Daniel Fast.

—H. MILLER

Drink Up!

If anyone thirsts, let him come to me and drink.
Rivers of living water will brim and spill out of the depths of anyone
who believes in me this way, just as the Scripture says.
—John 7:37-38 MSG

As soon I got out of bed and my feet hit the floor this morning, I headed straight for the kitchen to get a drink of water. I woke up feeling parched, and satisfying my thirst was all I could think about. I didn't just sip the water, either. I gulped it down as quickly as I could, and I felt so much better after I did.

Water is essential to life, and our bodies must have adequate amounts of it to thrive. All you have to do is type in "benefits of water" on any internet search engine, and you'll find hundreds of reasons why it's important to drink the water your body needs. One way water helps us as we fast is by removing toxins. Toxins are poisonous substances that cause damage to the body, resulting in all kinds of illness and health problems.

Our souls also need hydration, refreshing streams of living water that only Jesus can bring to our thirsty lives. Jesus promises that "whoever drinks of the water that I will give him will never be thirsty again. The water that I will give him will become in him a spring of water welling up

Verses for additional study:
Psalm 1:2 – 3
John 4:7 – 15
John 6:35
John 7:37 – 38

The Daniel Fast was an incredible journey for us. Neither my husband nor I had ever fasted before, so it was a totally new road for us to travel. Once I got through the first few days and changed my way of thinking, I was able to switch my focus from what I could and couldn't eat to the true reason I was fasting.

I really grew in my relationship with God and learned to lean on him for strength in a whole new way. I now fast on a regular basis and am always amazed at what God does.

— M. DAY

to eternal life" (John 4:14 ESV). Only the Lord can satisfy our deepest longings. Only he can flush out the toxins of anger, bitterness, jealousy, unforgiveness, and rebellion. Only Jesus, our Savior, can cleanse us from the inside out.

Every time you drink a glass of water during your fast, let it be a reminder that Jesus is your Living Water. He has unlimited stores of blessing, peace, power, and wisdom to pour into your life. Drink deeply of the Lord today. Find delight in the truth of his Word. Thirst for him alone.

Lord, I'm thirsty for you and your Word. Nothing satisfies but you. Fill me up today so that my life overflows with your love.

DAY 5

The Breath of Life

The Spirit of God has made me;
the breath of the Almighty gives me life.
— Job 33:4

One day I found myself struggling to explain to my daughters that even though we can't see Jesus and feel his arms around us, he is a real person. After discussing this concept for a few minutes, my six-year-old, Isabelle, finally said, "Mommy, I get it. Jesus is an air person."

Isabelle was simply stating what is obvious to her: she can't see Jesus with her eyes, but she knows he's there. And she's exactly right. Jesus *is* a real person, not some imaginary friend or a fictional character in a story. He's as real as the air we breathe. Just as our bodies are not able to survive without oxygen, we cannot live apart from Christ. Oh, we can exist just fine, but without him our lives are meaningless and empty.

I don't ever want to forget what my life was like before Jesus saved me. I was dead in my sins, without hope and without God. I was headed down a path to destruction. But one summer day more than thirty years ago, God rescued me from the kingdom of darkness and made me alive in Christ. He also implanted his Holy Spirit into my heart so that I would never be away from his presence.

Verses for additional study:
Ephesians 1:13
Ephesians 2:1, 4–5, 12
Romans 5:5
Romans 8:26

If you know the Lord, his Spirit lives in you. Your eyes may not see him, but he is there. This precious gift, who is also your Comforter, Counselor, Intercessor, Teacher, and Friend, is always with you, breathing his life into you so you can truly live.

God, thank you for giving me life, both physically and spiritually, and for sending your Holy Spirt to live in me so I would never be alone.

For about a year, I resisted the Holy Spirit's nudges to engage in a time of prayer and fasting. When our pastor asked our church to consider participating in a Daniel Fast, I immediately knew I needed to do it.

On top of praying for our church, I also prayed for family members who needed God to intervene in some tough situations. Did God answer? Yes, but not right away. God is so faithful and does more than we could even think or imagine! I am so blessed to have had the opportunity to obey the leading of the Spirit by fasting for my church and family. I believe my obedience allowed me to participate in God's answer to these prayers.

— R. ENKE

Cries in the Night

> The LORD is gracious and compassionate,
> slow to anger and rich in love.
> —Psalm 145:8

Last night was a very long night. My daughter ran into the bathroom nearly every hour to get sick, and I got up with her. Each time I was awakened, though, it became harder to get out of bed. As I pulled the covers off to get up for the fifth or sixth time, I reminded myself, "*Compassion,* Kristen. Be patient and compassionate."

At 4:30 a.m., I decided to just stay up and try to do some work on the computer. Almost as soon as I started writing, I heard Isabelle dry-heaving, so I went into the bathroom. In a shaky voice, she said, "I just want you with me." She was scared and wanted the comfort of having me close. I gave her a kiss on the top of her head and put my arms around her while she threw up. After she finished, I washed her face, tucked her back into bed, and prayed for her.

As I was cleaning up the bathroom, I couldn't help thinking about how the Lord responds to us in our time of need. Isaiah 30:18 says, "The LORD longs to be gracious to you; he rises to show you compassion." Our

Verses for additional study:
Psalm 116:5
Psalm 145:8 – 9
2 Corinthians 1:3
Colossians 3:12
1 Peter 3:8

We started the fast specifically to be in prayer for God's direction regarding orphan ministry and/or adoption. The day before the fast was over, God showed me that we need to follow him into Sierra Leone, Africa. We are already sponsoring children there, and I am planning a trip to visit and help in the orphanage. I feel very strongly that this will be a long-term ministry for our family and may lead to adoption. I believe with all my heart that this fast is what led to our vision and peacefulness about where we are headed! — J. WIDHALM

loving Father doesn't hesitate when we call out to him. He is always ready to come to our rescue.

No matter what you're going through, whether you're sick or lonely or scared, your gracious God is listening. As soon as your desperate cries reach his ears, he will surround you with his unconditional love and mercy. You can find comfort in God's promise that he will never leave you nor forsake you, which means you won't ever have to go through anything alone. When you find yourself facing the darkest of nights, cry out to the Lord, and find strength in his presence. He is waiting to help you.

Father, thank you for being a God of compassion and for always being there when I pray. Open my eyes to practical ways I can show your compassion to others.

DAY 7

A Good Work

He who began a good work in you will carry it
on to completion until the day of Christ Jesus.
—*Philippians 1:6*

Nehemiah had a successful career as cupbearer to the king, yet deep within him, he sensed the Lord calling him toward something different. Something radical. Something only God could do.

The task seemed monumental and impossible. The walls of Jerusalem were broken down, leaving the people defenseless against attack. Nehemiah knew that God wanted him to leave the comfort of palace life to lead his people in rebuilding the city walls.

Nehemiah responded in faith and obedience. He fasted and prayed. He boldly requested permission from the king and for his help in getting supplies. He wisely examined the condition of the walls before beginning reconstruction. He started the work.

From day one, Nehemiah and God's people endured intense persecution. Their enemies ridiculed and mocked them, hoping that they would give up. But the Israelites kept working day after day with all of their

Verses for additional study:

Nehemiah 1:4
Nehemiah 2:4 – 9,
    11 – 15, 20
Nehemiah 4:6
Nehemiah 6:15 – 16
Psalm 138:8

hearts, believing that the Lord would give them success. As a result, the massive city walls of Jerusalem were completed in record time. When the surrounding nations heard that the walls were completed in just fifty-two days, they were afraid and lost their self-confidence, because they realized that the work had been done with the help of God.

God calls each of us to a great work. Like Nehemiah and the Israelites, we undoubtedly will face fierce opposition. When the enemy hurls accusations our way and tries to defeat us, we can stand our ground on the truth of God's Word. I love Nehemiah's response to his enemies' relentless attempts to distract him: "I am carrying on a great project and cannot go down" (6:3). He refused to be shaken and remained focused on the purposes of God. We must remember that just as God was faithful in helping his people to rebuild the walls of Jerusalem, he will also complete the good work he has begun in our lives.

I quit my job with a CPA firm to go out on my own and just work a few hours a week. Three months went by, and while I was making some money, it seemed like we were always struggling. I considered getting a part-time job, but my husband said he felt like God had something else for me. Deep down, I knew he was right.

During the Daniel Fast, we prayed for direction with my business, and the Thursday before the Daniel Fast ended, the Lord opened up the windows of heaven and poured business and clients into our lives! God answered us in a mighty way, and we don't believe that we would have gotten that clear of an answer if we hadn't been on the Daniel Fast.
— T. Yearack

God, you have a plan for my life, and I am confident that you will bring it to completion as I surrender to you. I refuse to be distracted by the enemy and thrown off course by his wicked schemes. My eyes are on you, Sovereign Lord, to finish the good work you have started in me.

Congratulations! You made it through your first week! How are you doing so far? God is working in you and all around you. Continue to trust the Lord for strength to persevere. As you begin week 2, remember Philippians 4:13. You can do it!

When Affliction Is Good

It was good for me to be afflicted
so that I might learn your decrees.
—*Psalm 119:71*

A few years ago, I experienced major problems with my skin when the eczema I'd dealt with since childhood became increasingly worse. I tried everything—topical creams, oral and topical steroids, anti-inflammatory medications, and even light therapy. Most days I walked around in a zombie-like state, exhausted from the itching and scratching that kept me awake at night. I was irritable, depressed, and didn't feel like myself at all. I was so miserable in my own skin that I knew I'd have a breakdown if I didn't experience some relief.

Verses for additional study:
Psalm 119:68,
  75 – 76, 143
Psalm 145:17

During this dark season, the Lord led me to Psalm 119:71, which says, "It was good for me to be afflicted so that I might learn your decrees." I thought, "Good? There's nothing *good* about this, Lord! I look and feel horrible. I'm tired of dealing with this problem, and I don't understand how anything about it could be good." However, instead of continuing the pity party, I began to meditate on other verses in that same chapter that reminded me of God's goodness and faithfulness, which remain unchanged despite any trials he may allow into my life.

Slowly, my mind and heart were transformed as I viewed my situation from God's perspective. I learned to lean on the Lord for strength. I developed a passion for his Word. I prayed more often and with greater fervency. I realized that my skin problems weren't a punishment from the Lord but a way to learn how to focus on him as my source of strength and comfort. He allowed me to experience those physical challenges not because he was upset with me but because he loved me. He redeemed that particular trial, painful as it was, by drawing me closer to him.

After years of struggling with my weight, the Lord brought several things across my path, one of which was the Daniel Fast. The first day was easy! I was so excited and willing to give everything to him. By day three, I was ready to quit! God spoke to me, though, and let me know that quitting when things get hard is what I had done so many times in the past, and all it had gotten me was more than a hundred pounds overweight. I decided to continue the fast.

Over the course of my twenty-one-day fast, I lost seven pounds. But more than that, I learned that I can finish something and that I *can* do *all* things through Christ, who gives me strength. I will lose the extra weight, and it will all be to his glory!   — M. GIVLER

Are you going through a difficult time in your life that you don't understand? Are you weary from the struggle, and do you wonder what God's purpose might be? Good news: you don't have to understand why it's happening; *you only need to trust him.* The Lord is working this problem out for the good, even if you can't see it right now, and he will use whatever it takes to transform you into the image of Christ. Embrace his precious promises, and ask him to give you a special verse that will strengthen your faith. Someday soon you'll look back on this trial, reflect on all that God has done, and be able to say, "It was good for me to be afflicted."

God, I know that there is purpose in the pain of affliction. Keep me from sinking into despair when trials come. I want to bring honor and glory to you, no matter what the circumstances are in my life.

Be Patient, and Don't Grumble!

DAY
9

Give thanks in all circumstances,
for this is God's will for you in Christ Jesus.
—1 Thessalonians 5:18

Having my garbage disposal explode all over the kitchen isn't exactly an example of enduring suffering, but it certainly was a test of patience. The remnants of apples, beets, and oranges blanketed my hardwood floor. It was a mess ... a chunky, bright-red mess.

Verses for additional study:
Psalm 7:17
Psalm 28:7
Psalm 118:28

As I cleaned up the kitchen, I felt anxious and stressed. I thought about all the things I had to do and how this wasn't the way I wanted to start my day. I was angry. I silently chastised my husband for not making the seal tighter when he put the sink back together a few weeks ago. I was irritated that my daughters kept asking when I was going to make them breakfast. Wasn't it obvious I had a disaster on my hands?

In that moment, two verses came to mind: "Be patient" (James 5:7) and "Don't grumble" (James 5:9).

Uh oh. I was clearly guilty on both counts. I was certainly complaining in my spirit, and I didn't have a single ounce of patience in me. Determined not to let this unexpected incident ruin my day, I stopped, took a deep breath, and asked God to give me strength. Not only did he help me clean up the food flung all over my kitchen but also he gave me what I needed the most — his perspective. God reminded me that trials of every shape and size, even the most unpleasant ones, are often heaven-sent opportunities to mature as a follower of Christ. I realized that the garbage-disposal fiasco that morning was an opportunity to put my faith into action by being thankful, despite the inconvenience of it all.

As you go about your day today, view any challenging situations you face as ways to be more like Jesus. When you see the circumstances in your life through God's eyes, you won't be rattled when your plans are interrupted. You won't grumble and complain. You will respond with a thankful heart.

Lord God, I know trials are part of life and that you use them to help me grow. Help me to give thanks in all circumstances.

We decided to do a Daniel Fast after putting our house on the market. Within fifteen days of the listing, we had an offer. By day sixteen of placing our house on the market and day twelve of our fast, we had a signed contract. We knew this was God's doing, as the housing market is still not that great, and the first week the house was listed, there was ice and snow on the ground and very cold temperatures. The Daniel Fast was amazing for us, and I am forever changed by my experience.

— A. Gannon

DAY
10

Tunnel Vision

Since God so loved us, we also ought to love one another.
No one has ever seen God; but if we love one another,
God lives in us and his love is made complete in us.
—1 John 4:11 – 12

Verses for additional study:
Matthew 22:37 – 39
Philippians 2:3 – 4
1 Peter 4:8

I recently had one of those mornings when I woke up feeling irritable and groggy. I had a massive headache and felt like I'd been hit by a train. All morning long, I carried around a "woe is me" attitude. After a few hours of this self-inflicted misery, I finally sat down and opened my Bible to 1 John 4:7 – 16, the passage in which the apostle John writes so eloquently about God's love for us and how we are to love one another.

My whole outlook changed within a matter of minutes. I no longer felt sorry for myself. In fact, I wasn't even thinking about myself at all. Instead, my heart was lifted and encouraged as I thought about God and his amazing love.

God's love is mind-boggling. It's hard to understand why he chooses to pour out his grace and mercy upon such imperfect, stubborn, and rebellious people. But, thankfully, he does! God loved us so much that he sent his Son, Jesus, as a sacrifice for our sins. Jesus' death on the cross made it possible for us to experience the full extent of God's love. However, this love isn't given to us for our enjoyment alone. God pours his love into our lives so that we might share it with others.

I closed my Bible and realized what my real problem was. I had a severe case of tunnel vision. Tunnel vision, from a medical standpoint, is the loss of peripheral vision — or side vision — which means we see only what is directly in front of us. Just because I didn't feel well, I'd lost all ability to see anyone else's needs. My gaze was limited to me, myself, and I.

Even though my headache didn't go away for several hours, my vision improved immediately after reading the truth of God's Word. He showed me that it's impossible to love people when I can't even see them. And to see them, I have to stop focusing on myself.

When life gets you down and you feel your vision narrowing, spend a few minutes with God. Turn your attention to him. Your peripheral vision will return, and you'll be free to share God's love with those around you.

Father, it's easy to get so wrapped up in my own life that I become oblivious to the needs of the people around me. Help me to humble myself so that I can share your life-changing love.

During the fast, I really sought the Lord's direction for ministry. I have a passion for youth but wasn't sure where God wanted me to serve. One day my son went on a field trip and picked up a brochure he thought I would like. It was information on gangs. As I read the brochure, my heart broke for those kids. Then it hit me — I needed be involved in urban youth ministry.

I told the Lord I would go wherever he wanted to take me, even if it meant uprooting and moving my whole family. Before the fast, that was a big *no way.* We did move, and God has opened up a whole new mission field for us among friends and family members. My new job, which is in the "bad area" of town, puts me right in the thick of gang activity. Murders are frequent, and most of them are gang related. Despite these challenges, we are seeing God at work. I wouldn't have experienced any of these blessings if I hadn't been listening to God through prayer and fasting.

—D. Oltman

Dry Bones

I am the LORD, the God of all mankind.
Is anything too hard for me?
—*Jeremiah 32:27*

A few years ago, I took an anatomy class. I guess I should clarify that it wasn't a regular anatomy class. It was *gross* anatomy, which means we worked on human cadavers.

One particular memory from that class will always stay with me. As I stood over a cadaver, I thought about the fact that the only difference between the body of the woman lying on the table and me was life. All of the parts were there — her muscles, tissues, and bones — but her spirit was gone. In that moment, I was struck by the fact that God is the one who breathes life into us, and without his Spirit indwelling our hearts, we are dead inside.

The prophet Ezekiel also had an unforgettable encounter with a set of bones. The Lord led him to a valley that was covered with them and asked, "Son of man, can these bones live?" (Ezek. 37:3). Notice that the Lord doesn't say, "Are these bones *alive*?" It is quite obvious they aren't. They are dead. All dried up. Useless.

> The Daniel Fast was an awesome experience for us. My husband's business was facing its worst year yet financially. He had lost clients and income because of the economy and other situations. During the fast, we prayed for God to bring new clients, and God delivered! He replaced all the lost income, and then some. It was a very special time with the Lord. Through our fasting and praying, God not only changed our circumstances; he also changed our walk with him. I can't wait to see what else God will do as we fast and seek him!
>
> — D. CHRONISTER

Ezekiel isn't too sure where the Lord is going with his line of questioning, so he plays it safe and says, "O Sovereign LORD, you alone know" (v. 3). Ezekiel doesn't answer the Lord's question with a bold and confident yes because he can't see beyond the natural process of death so clearly evident before him. His perspective is limited. However, the Lord doesn't condemn Ezekiel for his lack of faith. Instead, in his love and mercy, he gives Ezekiel a vision of what can happen when God enters a seemingly hopeless situation.

Verses for additional study:
Job 33:4
Proverbs 14:30
Romans 4:17

The Lord tells Ezekiel to prophesy to the bones, to command them to come to life. As Ezekiel speaks, he hears a rattling sound. The bones are moving! They come together, one by one. Flesh and tendons appear; skin covers them. However, the bodies are still dead.

Again the Lord tells Ezekiel to prophesy and to call forth the breath of life. When Ezekiel commands the breath to enter into the bodies, a vast army stands before him — hundreds of living, breathing human beings. Now Ezekiel can answer God's question with complete confidence: "Yes! These bones *can* live!"

Like Ezekiel, you may find yourself standing in the middle of a valley of dry bones. You can't see beyond what is right in front of you. God wants to change your viewpoint. Whatever you are facing may seem hopeless, but it's not. Whether it's a lifeless marriage, a dead-end job, or an uncertain future, the Lord wants to speak life into your situation. Put your trust in his Word, and watch the God of the universe do amazing things.

God, I put my trust in you today. Even when situations in my life seem hopeless, I know that nothing is too difficult for you!

The Right Tool

> Your word is a lamp to guide my feet
> and a light for my path.
> — *Psalm 119:105 NLT*

My husband is a tool man through and through. If something around the house is broken and needs repairing, he feels giddy, rather than inconvenienced. He immediately drops what he's doing, bolts to the man cave, and digs through his arsenal of contraptions, gadgets, and thingamajigs in search of just the right tool for the job.

He relishes the process of restoration, making whatever has been damaged whole again. Focused on the task at hand, he refuses to give up if problems occur along the way. However, there are moments when he emerges from the toolshed feeling frustrated and incompetent because he can't find what he needs to finish the work. Progress is halted until the proper tool is located.

Verses for additional study:
Psalm 19:8
Psalm 119:11, 33 – 35
Proverbs 6:23

How do you respond when something in your life breaks and needs to be repaired? Do problems prompt anger, or are you able to receive them with a sense of anticipation? James 1:2 – 4 shows us how trials can benefit us: "When troubles come your way, consider it an opportunity for great joy. For you know that when your faith is tested, your endurance has a chance to grow. So let it grow, for when your endurance is fully developed, you will be perfect and complete, needing nothing" (NLT).

When struggles come our way, we don't ever lack the right tool for the job. We have one multipurpose tool — the Word of God — which is capable of guiding us through every repair job we encounter. The Bible is both a lamp and a light, which means that it shines brightly into our circumstances as well as illuminates the steps we should take. If we embrace this powerful tool God has given us, we will experience peace and hope, even during the most difficult challenges of life. Because, in the words of my handyman husband, "Having the right tool makes all the difference."

Lord God, your powerful Word holds the answers for every problem or situation in my life. Help me to discipline myself to read it daily. I want to saturate my mind with your truth so I can be strong in you.

When Kristen first shared the idea of a Daniel Fast, I wondered how it could benefit us as a church and as individuals. Well, I must say that I was pleasantly surprised.

After going through our first fast of twenty-one days in January, my wife and I can say that it was a great blessing in our lives personally, and I believe we will be seeing the long-term results at our church. It's amazing how focused you can become during a fast. I believe this could become a unifying experience for our entire church family, so we plan to call a Daniel Fast at the beginning of next year.

— Pastor D. Mercaldo

DAY
13

Fear

Do not fear, for I am with you; do not be dismayed,
for I am your God. I will strengthen you and help you;
I will uphold you with my righteous right hand.
— *Isaiah 41:10*

Verses for additional study:
Psalm 27:1
Psalm 56:3
Isaiah 26:3
Romans 8:15
2 Timothy 1:7

Isabelle wasn't coming down without a fight. Our six-year-old had just climbed a thirty-five-foot rock face like a seasoned pro. She had no problem navigating the various rock formations, easily finding a handhold here, a foothold there. Avid rock climbers, my husband and I were beaming with pride when she did it all by herself. Once she got to the top, her dad talked her through what she needed to do to come back down to the ground. She had done it at least a dozen times in the past, so we were confident she would descend easily without a problem.

Suddenly, though, her foot slipped. She spun around, slammed her elbow against the rock wall, and ended up dangling in the air. All I heard was her bloodcurdling scream. Actually, it was a series of screams. I don't think I've ever seen her so panicked.

We tried to calm her down, but it was no use. Nothing we said got through to her. Between sobs, she cried out, "I'm scared! I can't do it! My elbow hurts! I don't know what to do!" She was paralyzed with fear and determined to stay right where she was until her father came to her rescue.

It was very frustrating for me to see my daughter struggle, especially when she didn't have to. I tried to remain patient and loving, but after several unsuccessful attempts to coax her down, I began to get angry. Why wouldn't she let us help her? Didn't she trust us? Couldn't she see we weren't going to let her fall?

Eventually, my husband climbed up to her. At first, Isabelle didn't even want his help and refused to move toward him. Stubborn girl. Eventually, though, she took her father's hand and slowly made her way to the ground. She cried the whole way down.

As we drove home, I thought about how often I am just like Isabelle. Many times I'm hanging out on the side of a mountain in my life, white-knuckled with worry and fear. All I can think about are the what-ifs: What if I can't do it? What if I make a mistake? What if I get hurt? I cry out to God for his help, but when he reaches out to me, I resist. Yet the Lord is always the perfect parent. He doesn't chastise or condemn. He simply waits patiently until I get my act together. If I refuse to submit and remain in rebellion, he comes to my rescue. He brings me back to himself, even if I kick and scream all the way.

God loves us and wants the best for us. All we have to do is trust him. Our Father has a tight grip and won't ever let us go.

Lord, because you are with me, I have nothing to fear. Thank you for giving me strength when I am weak. You are my Rock, and I put my trust in you.

I work in the world of Wall Street, a difficult place to be in because of all the economic turmoil that has plagued us in recent years. It's hard to feel peaceful when I'm afraid my livelihood could disappear at any moment. I prayed for the Lord to guide me and take hold of every facet of my life. I gave *everything* — my problems, my job, my money, my family, my life, and my health — to God. This happened around the same time my church challenged us to do the Daniel Fast. I love to eat, especially all the wrong foods, so I knew this would be difficult for me. I was challenged. I did it, nonetheless, and felt closer to the Lord in fulfilling the pledge. I have found renewed vigor and love for Jesus and have rededicated my life to him.

— M. Quan

Run!

Let us run with perseverance
the race marked out for us.
—*Hebrews 12:1*

*Verses for
additional study:*
2 Corinthians 12:9
Hebrews 12:1
2 Timothy 4:7

Running doesn't come naturally to me. I definitely wouldn't call myself a runner, although I did compete in a few races as part of a track team way back in junior high. As soon as the starting gun was fired, I ran as fast as my little legs would take me. In shorter races, my all-out sprint worked great. However, when it came to the longer distances, I couldn't maintain that explosive pace and often fizzled out before crossing the finish line. I didn't know anything about running skills or technique and didn't know that I needed to pace myself. I just gave 100 percent every time.

Doing the Daniel Fast is like running a long-distance race. On day 1, you jumped out of the starting blocks, full of energy and determination. It's now day fourteen. How is your race going? Are you making strides, or are you losing steam?

At the beginning of the year, I felt strongly that God was calling us to do the Daniel Fast. My wife had done the fast the year before, but I chose not to participate because it seemed to be more than I could take on. However, this time something was different. I was confident that God was going to give me the grace to do the fast.

The first two days, I had caffeine-withdrawal headaches. By the third day, though, the headaches stopped, and I had tremendous energy and focus. Three weeks went by and we were done. I can't say that I was miraculously changed, but I can say that I felt a million miles closer to God, my wife, and my purpose in life. It was the most productive fasting experience I've ever had.

— W. AXTELL

If you're feeling strong, then keep up the good pace. However, if you're wondering why you signed up for this event, don't slow down! Now is not the time to let up. Now is the time to refuel, refocus, and recharge!

The Lord has called you to this fast, and he will sustain you. Do whatever you need to do to spend more time with him in prayer. Adjust your schedule to make it happen, and don't make excuses or allow yourself to become distracted. This race is far too important. Then in a week when you cross the finish line, you will be able to say, "I have fought the good fight, I have finished the race, I have kept the faith" (2 Tim. 4:7). *That's* the kind of running that pleases the Lord. That's the kind of running that wins.

Lord God, I will keep praying, reading your Word, adhering to the food guidelines, and trusting in you each day of this fast. Thank you for helping me to persevere, even when it gets tough. Your strength will carry me so that I can finish strong.

Two down, one to go! As you finish your second week, stay motivated and strong. Don't "check out" before the fast is completed. Yes, you have made it through two weeks, which is great, but you still have one week left. Keep trusting in the Lord for the strength you need to fulfill your commitment. He still has work to do!

Follow the Cloud

> At the LORD's command they encamped,
> and at the LORD's command they set out.
> —*Numbers 9:23*

I love to go camping with my family, but what I don't like is getting everything together — the sleeping bags, the air mattress (yes, we're all about comfort), the food, the clothes, and everything else necessary to survive a few nights in a tent. By the time our car is loaded up, my neck muscles are so tight it usually takes me several miles to relax. Although all the stress of going camping is worth it once we get out in nature, I could easily do without the packing part.

Verses for additional study:
Numbers 9:15 – 23
Deuteronomy 13:4
Psalm 38:15
Psalm 130:5

The Israelites knew all about the challenges of camping. Their forty-year expedition in the wilderness was certainly no vacation. As nomads, they were without permanent homes and lived in tents in the desert.

In addition to their personal belongings, the Israelites also traveled with the tabernacle, which was the portable dwelling place for God's presence. During this time, the Lord provided a sign to the Israelites — a cloud — to assure them that he was with them. Whenever the cloud lifted above the tabernacle, the people knew it was time to move on. However, when the cloud stood still, they set up camp and remained there until the cloud lifted again. Sometimes the cloud hovered over the tabernacle from evening until the next morning. Other times it stayed for a month or longer. The Israelites didn't know when they would go or where they would be going. They had absolutely no control or say in the matter. They lived day by day in complete dependence on the guidance of the Lord. And yet, despite the uncertainty and inconvenience of this lifestyle, they obeyed.

Where are you in your journey with the Lord? Are you camping out and waiting for the Lord's instructions? Are you on the move, following in the direction God is leading you? Wherever you are, know that the Lord is with you. Listen to his voice. If God says wait, then sit tight. If he says go, then start packing. Be like the Israelites. Follow where God leads.

Dear God, I know you have a plan for my life. You have work for me to do and places for me to go. As I spend time in prayer and in your Word, speak to my heart. Show me if now is a time to move or a time to wait on you.

I sat in shock one February afternoon after hearing my principal say, "The school board may not renew your contract next year." I couldn't believe it. Only three years earlier, God had led me to the school where I now teach and hadn't given any clear indication that my time there would be ending.

I resolved to seek the Lord through a Daniel Fast for direction in my career. God gave me Psalm 37:7 at the start of my fast: "Be still before the LORD and wait patiently for him." I wish I could say the board voted in my favor, but they didn't. I trust that this situation is part of the larger plan God has to work everything together for the good. The biggest thing God gave me during the fast was supernatural peace. It's a peace that continues to flow as he directs me to wait. It's hard to do sometimes, but I am waiting with a sense of awe and expectation for what lies ahead. I am so thankful to serve a God who assures me the best is yet to come!

—D. PEACHEY

DAY 16

Stop Being So Stubborn!

Do not be stubborn ...
but submit yourselves to the LORD.
—*2 Chronicles 30:8 NLT*

Verses for additional study:
Hosea 4:16
Psalm 25:9
Psalm 81:10 – 14
James 4:10

As our two girls were getting ready for school one day, I overheard my six-year-old, Isabelle, say in frustration, "This backpack is being so *stubborn*!" Jocelyn, my four-year-old daughter, was puzzled and asked, "What does *stubborn* mean?" I couldn't wait to hear the perspective of my six-year-old, who has a bit of a stubborn streak herself. After a few seconds, Isabelle replied, "It's wanting to do things your own way." I was so taken aback by her answer and the fact that she had that amount of insight at such a young age.

Even though people sometimes make jokes about being hardheaded, stubbornness is not a trait to be proud of. Many verses in the Bible warn of the danger of being arrogant or stiff-necked. The Bible makes it clear that refusing to listen to God and following our own inclinations has serious consequences: "But my people would not listen to me. They kept doing whatever they wanted, following the stubborn desires of their evil hearts. They went backward instead of forward" (Jeremiah 7:24 NLT). Being stubborn not only stunts spiritual growth; it moves our lives in the wrong direction!

The first step to softening a stubborn, arrogant heart is to submit — to release your desire for control and say to the Lord, "Whatever you want is what I want." That requires throwing pride out the window and humbling yourself.

By fasting and denying myself, I found that God opened my eyes to areas in my life that I've been avoiding. When I was still and listened to what God had to say, he showed me the work I needed to do. I also learned that I can deny myself and reap rewards that I never could have imagined. Would I do the fast again? Yes, without hesitation.

— A. Stillings

Father, there are times when my need for control causes me to be prideful, arrogant, and downright stubborn. Help me to learn to submit instead of insisting on having my own way. I follow after you, for you are my Good Shepherd, and I know I am safe in your care.

Above, Not Below

Set your minds on things above,
not on earthly things.
—*Colossians 3:2*

As I tucked my daughter into bed the other night, I noticed her Bible lying on top of her comforter near her feet. When I asked her why she put it there, she said she needed to keep it close so she could read it as soon as she woke up in the morning.

No wonder the Lord said that we need to have the faith of a little child when it comes to the kingdom of heaven! I want to be like my daughter, so excited about being with the Lord that I can't wait to spend time with him as soon as I get up. Too often, though, my mind is swarming with all the things that need to get done that day. Instead of resting in the Lord, I get stressed. Before I even walk out the door, I'm overwhelmed. Even

Verses for additional study:
Matthew 18:1 – 4
Philippians 4:8

though I may read the Bible and pray, I'm unable to receive what God wants to show me because I'm distracted.

But on those mornings when my eyes are on the Lord, I'm filled with peace. My first waking thoughts are on the Lord, and I can't wait to sit at his feet. As I open the Word and read about God's love for me, my heart is full. My worries are all forgotten as I spend time in the Lord's presence.

First Corinthians 2:16 says that we have the mind of Christ, which means that the Holy Spirit gives us spiritual understanding and the ability to obey God's command. We set our minds on things above — spiritual, eternal matters — by spending time meditating on truth. Each verse we read or memorize works to transform our thoughts to keep them from being consumed with earthly, temporal concerns.

> My husband and I have been doing a Daniel Fast in January for the past several years. A few years ago, we used our fast specifically to discern whether God was prompting us to move from our current work into a senior pastorate position. By the end of the fast, we both knew it was time to resign our positions and trust that the Lord would show us the way to go. We moved back to Canada and became the new pastors at a church in Ontario. I will always remember how God used the Daniel Fast to give us the direction we needed.
>
> — C. Johnston

What is your mindset today? Be determined to maintain an upward focus by being consistent in your study of God's Word. If you find yourself feeling weighed down with matters of things below, open up the Bible to direct your thoughts upward once again.

Lord God, I set my mind on your truth and refuse to let anxiety invade my thoughts. I will rest in your perfect peace today as I remember your promises to me.

DAY 18

Desire the Prize

I press on toward the goal to win the prize
for which God has called me heavenward in Christ Jesus.
— *Philippians 3:14*

It was early in the morning, still dark outside, and rain was pelting my windshield. Trucks were staggered along the side of the highway like mile markers. Even though the weather was nasty and cold, I could easily see the bright orange parkas in the distance as two men walked toward the woods. "Those guys are nuts!" I thought. Only one thing could lead them to go deer hunting in that kind of weather when it would have been much easier to stay in bed. They were motivated by desire. Pure desire.

I had to admit, I admired their commitment. Those hunters had their eyes on the prize of bringing home a deer, a reward they considered to be worth every minute of discomfort they might have to endure.

As I drove along, I thought about what it takes to seek the Lord with that kind of passion. It requires persevering through the storms of life and remaining committed to the Lord. It could mean getting up early in the morning to do your Bible study, maybe even before the sun comes up. It might involve an illness that causes you to depend upon the Lord in a way you've never known before. What I realized is that strong affection for the Lord begins with a desire to do whatever it takes to grow closer to him.

Verses for additional study:
Psalm 40:8
Psalm 73:25
1 Corinthians 9:24

Are you seeking the Lord with that kind of passion? If not, why not? Refuse to let apathy and laziness set in. Don't hit the snooze button on life and crawl back under the covers. Your time on earth is short, so make the most of every day you're given. Press on, my friend. Desire Jesus more than anything or anyone else. He is your prize. There is no greater reward.

Lord Jesus, you truly are my reason for living. I desire you more than anything else. Give me a greater passion for you and your Word. I long to know you more.

Our entire family of five — yes, even three teenagers — agreed to do the Daniel Fast together. We fasted and prayed about decisions facing our church, and we also prayed for a new home. God moved miraculously on both accounts. Our Wilsons Creek Campus launch was wildly successful with more than 2,100 people attending the grand opening, and God gave us the very home for which we had prayed the previous year. Prayer and fasting really do work! — PASTOR C. COOK

The Aroma of Christ

Live in love as Christ also loved us.
He gave his life for us as an offering and sacrifice,
a soothing aroma to God.
—*Ephesians 5:2 GW*

You've probably heard the saying, "You are what you eat." Here's one, though, that may be new to you: "You smell like what you eat."

Garlic is one of my favorite herbs because it adds a unique, distinctive zip to any dish. Just think of what pesto would be without garlic. Bland and boring. Spaghetti sauce? I can't imagine it without a clove or two. Garlic not only tastes good, but it's also a natural antibiotic and is beneficial to the body. Regular intake of garlic may be effective in lowering cholesterol levels, fighting the common cold, and reducing the risk of certain cancers. It can also be used as a mosquito repellant!

However, too much garlic can cause mild stomach distress, such as indigestion and bloating. The worst side effects, though, are what others around you are forced to endure — your bad breath and foul body odor. The sulfuric compounds of garlic contribute to its sharp taste and strong smell, which remain in your system and hang around with you for days after eating it.

On a positive note, there are some foods that help to decrease natural body odors, leaving us with a more pleasant scent: cardamom, cinnamon, cloves, nutmeg, fresh produce, and fresh, pure citrus juices.

As believers in Jesus, we carry a fragrance with us wherever we go, and it's up to us whether that fragrance is pleasant or repulsive. Just as some foods cause us to smell a particular way, our thoughts do as well. If we feed on lies, negative attitudes and behaviors come out, much like how garlic seeps through our pores when we sweat. Others are nauseated by our presence, and our aroma drives them away. People who don't know the Lord may be so put off by our offensive odor that they turn away from God and never get a taste of his salvation.

To carry a pleasant scent, we must ingest the truth of the Word. As people inhale the sweet-smelling scents of God's love in us, they are drawn to the Lord.

When people take a whiff of you, do they smell something sweet or stinky? You are the aroma of Christ to the world around you. Share his exquisite fragrance with someone today.

Verses for additional study:
John 13:34
2 Corinthians 2:14 – 16

Lord God, as I feed on your Word each day, fill me with your love so that my life is an attractive aroma that brings people closer to you.

When I started my first Daniel Fast, I didn't know what to expect, but I was excited to see how God would work in my life. My primary prayer focus during the fast was my upcoming marriage. My fiancée and I wanted supernatural wisdom to guide us through all the decisions we needed to make, which included everything from the wedding details to financial issues. Rather than becoming worried or anxious, we sought direction from the Lord through the Daniel Fast. Looking back, I can see how he paved the way for us by creating a smooth transition into our new life together. I give all credit to the Lord! — J. Hardy

Content

Keep your lives free from the love of money
and be content with what you have.
—*Hebrews 13:5*

My two-week obsession with moving began after reading an article about how every serious writer should have a dedicated work space. Suddenly my laptop on the kitchen table seemed unprofessional and inadequate. The more I thought about it, the more convinced I was that I *needed* an office. I drove neighborhoods, looked up houses online, called and met with our realtor, and made plans to put our house on the market. It was exciting at first. However, it wasn't long before I felt overwhelmed.

Verses for additional study:
1 Timothy 6:6 – 11, 17
James 1:17

One day when I was vacuuming, I realized how much I really do love where we live. Even though there are moments when I wish we had more space, when it would be great to have a basement so the kids could run around and play, or to be able to write in my own office, I'm thankful for our home.

As believers in Jesus, we have many reasons to be satisfied because of what God has given us. After all, we have eternal life! Yet we struggle with feelings of discontentment, especially when we're bombarded with messages that tell us we need bigger, better, and more! Suddenly what we have isn't enough. Although there is nothing wrong with having nice worldly possessions, we shouldn't set our hearts on acquiring wealth. When we look to things to bring satisfaction and joy to our lives, we come up empty-handed every time.

God has provided everything you need for life and godliness through your knowledge of him. Your life is complete in the Lord. Be content. You don't lack anything if you know Jesus.

Lord, all that I truly need is found in you. Thank you for the countless ways you have blessed my life. Help me to remember that nothing in this world brings lasting contentment. Your love is the only source of true satisfaction and joy.

During my Daniel Fast, I focused on prayer for my finances. God showed me that even though I was praying about my situation, I wasn't fully surrendering my burdens to him. He knew that I was still feeling overwhelmed. After all, the Lord knows what is in our hearts. We can't hide anything from him. He comforted me through this verse: "Don't be afraid. Just stand still and watch the LORD rescue you today" (Exod. 14:13 NLT). I praise God and thank him for the assurance that he will rescue me. What an amazing God we serve!   — J. STOCKTON

Remember

Remember the wonders he has done.
— Psalm 105:5

Congratulations! You have made it to the final day of your Daniel Fast. I pray that your time with the Lord through prayer and fasting has truly surpassed anything you could have imagined.

As you finish your commitment, it's good to look back and remember how faithful the Lord has been. Reflect on all he has done — answered your prayers, given you strength, encouraged you through his Word, and sustained you through the power of his Holy Spirit. He has also given you a wonderful testimony. You have a unique story to tell about how God has worked in your life over the past three weeks.

One way you can record God's blessings is to journal about them. Write these things down now while they are still fresh in your mind. Another way is to share with someone how God answered a specific request that you prayed for during your fast. Also, I would love to hear

Verses for additional study:

Psalm 9:1 – 2
Psalm 40:5
Psalm 111:2 – 4
Psalm 145

your fasting testimony so I can post it on my blog (*www.ultimatedaniel fast.com*) to encourage others who are doing the Daniel Fast.

My prayer is that you will continue to pursue the Lord with the same frequency and fervency that you have known on your Daniel Fast. The Lord doesn't want your desire for him to wane just because your fast is completed. Now that you have tasted and seen that the Lord is good, aren't you hungry for more? May the Lord pour out his richest blessings on your life as you continue to hunger and thirst for him!

God did an amazing miracle in our lives through the Daniel Fast — he gave us our baby girl from Haiti. We had been trying to adopt for about two years, but nothing was working, and we were discouraged. One month after our fast ended, a woman from our church approached us about hosting a young Haitian girl who was to receive medical care in our area. She had been diagnosed with sickle-cell anemia, a devastating and incurable disease. We agreed, even though we knew it most likely would not turn into an adoption.

Long story short, when the doctors began treatment, they discovered that she didn't have the disease and is completely healthy. God healed her! Even though my husband and I are older than the age limit to adopt from Haiti, the government is making an exception and we are in the process of adopting her. It is truly a miracle in every way. God has been so good to us!

— J. Salazar

Lord God, I thank you for how you've blessed my life during this fast. You have been so good to me! Fill me with your power, Lord, and fan the flame you have begun in my heart. May my life shine so brightly for you that others are drawn to your great mercy and love. Great is your faithfulness, Lord God. I praise your holy name!

You did it. Three weeks ago, you had a goal — to pursue the Lord through the Daniel Fast — and now you are crossing the finish line in victory. God has heard every prayer and seen every struggle along the way, and he is pleased with how you ran the race. I pray that your time in the Word has increased your knowledge of truth, deepened your love for the Lord, and transformed you into a different person than you were twenty-one days ago. Praise God for all that he has done!

PART 3

the
FOOD

I ate no choice food; no meat or wine touched my lips …
until the three weeks were over.

—Daniel 10:3

Foods to Eat

- *Fruits:* fresh, frozen, dried, juiced, canned
- *Vegetables:* fresh, frozen, dried, juiced, canned
- *Whole grains:* amaranth, barley, brown rice, oats, quinoa, millet, whole wheat
- *Nuts and seeds:* almonds, cashews, macadamia nuts, peanuts, pecans, pine nuts, walnuts, pumpkin seeds, sesame seeds, sunflower seeds, nut butters
- *Unleavened bread:* whole grain breads made without yeast, sugars, or preservatives
- *Legumes (canned or dried):* black beans, black-eyed peas, cannellini beans, garbanzo beans (chickpeas), great northern beans, kidney beans, lentils, pinto beans, split peas
- *Quality oils:* canola, coconut, flaxseed, grapeseed, olive, peanut, sesame
- *Beverages:* distilled water, filtered water, spring water
- *Other:* herbs, spices, salt, pepper, seasonings, soy products, tofu

Foods to Avoid

- *Meat:* beef, buffalo, fish, lamb, pork, poultry
- *Dairy products:* butter, cheese, cream, eggs, milk
- *Sweeteners:* agave nectar, artificial sweeteners, cane juice, honey, molasses, raw sugar, granulated sugar, brown sugar, syrups, stevia
- *Leavened bread and yeast:* any bread with yeast, baked goods, Ezekiel bread (contains yeast and honey)
- *Refined and processed food products:* artificial flavorings, chemicals, food additives, preservatives, white flour, white rice
- *Deep-fried foods:* corn chips, French fries, potato chips
- *Solid fats:* lard, margarine, shortening
- *Beverages:* alcohol, caffeine, carbonated drinks, coffee, energy drinks, green tea, herbal tea, tea

Creating Your Daniel Fast Meal Plan

This section of the book contains more than one hundred recipes, and it provides at least one or two variations for each recipe, so you are equipped with an abundant supply of tasty meal possibilities for your Daniel Fast. However, since you probably have about as much free time to devote to meal planning as I do, I have provided a suggested basic Daniel Fast meal plan to get you started. (See pp. 65 – 67.) This plan consists of three weekly menus, each of which is divided into the following four recipe categories:

1. Breakfast
2. Appetizers and Snacks
3. Vegetables
4. Salads, Soups, and Main Dishes

Each category contains a pool of recipes from which you may choose. For example, using the pool of breakfast recipes listed in the suggested plan for week 1 (p. 65), you might decide that your Daniel Fast meal plan for breakfast during week 1 will look like this:

MONDAY: Nutty Fruit Cereal
TUESDAY: Nutty Fruit Cereal
WEDNESDAY: Strawberry-Banana Smoothie
THURSDAY: Baked Oatmeal
FRIDAY: Baked Oatmeal
SATURDAY: Nutty Fruit Cereal

Or your plan might look completely different! That's the best part about this plan; you are free to mix and match recipes, according to your likes and dislikes. It also gives you greater freedom in meal planning, instead of burdening you with a detailed menu for each day that's impossible to follow. The suggested recipes in each category are merely that — suggestions. You can always substitute another dish that you would like to try. There are plenty of tasty recipes in the book, so I say have at it! Refer to the index of recipes (p. 219) for ideas and check out my blog (*www.ultimatedanielfast.com*) to see mouthwatering photos of each dish.

If you decide to work from the suggested meal plans, refer to the "Daniel Fast Menu Planning Tool" in appendix 3 (p. 203) for further help in creating your meal plan and grocery shopping lists.

Week 1 Suggested Meal Plan

For a quick look at the ingredients for all of the recipes in this suggested meal plan, see pages 204–7.

Breakfast

Baked Oatmeal (p. 71)

Nutty Fruit Cereal (p. 77)

Strawberry-Banana Smoothie (p. 79)

Appetizers and Snacks

Broiled Polenta Squares (p. 83)

Cinnamon Roasted Almonds (p. 85)

Date Honey (p. 87)

Hummus (p. 92)

Trail Mix (p. 101)

Vegetables

Italian-Style Broccoli (p. 147)

Garlic Spring Peas with Leeks (p. 143)

Tarragon Roasted Asparagus (p. 157)

Salads, Soups, and Main Dishes

Mega Greek Salad (p. 106)

Fig, Pear, and Walnut Salad (p. 104)

Chunky Potato Soup (p. 124)

Tuscan Soup (p. 132)

Antipasto Pizza Pie (p. 160)

Black Bean Chili Bake (p. 161)

Romaine Wraps (p. 176)

Preparation Tips

- **Baked Oatmeal:** Make, but don't bake, up to two days before the fast begins. Store in refrigerator. Bake uncovered in the oven when you're ready to eat.
- **Cinnamon Roasted Almonds:** Use 1 cup in Trail Mix recipe.
- **Date Honey:** Make the day before your fast begins or on day 1.
- **Hummus:** Prepare and store in the refrigerator, or make a double batch and place half in the freezer to use later during your fast. Use to make Romaine Wraps.
- **Mega Greek Salad:** Save on salad assembly time at lunch or dinner by chopping vegetables earlier in the day so that they're ready to go.
- **Antipasto Pizza Pie:** Cook rice the night before or earlier in the day.
- **Black Bean Chili Bake:** Cook rice while you're preparing breakfast or lunch to speed up dinner preparation.

Week 1 Combinations to Try

Baked Oatmeal with Date Honey

Chunky Potato Soup with Tarragon Roasted Asparagus

Tuscan Soup with Fig, Pear, and Walnut Salad

Black Bean Chili Bake with Broiled Polenta Squares

Romaine Wraps with Tuscan Soup

Week 2 Suggested Meal Plan

For a quick look at the ingredients for all of the recipes in this suggested meal plan, see pages 208–12.

Breakfast

Coconut Fig Bars (p. 74)
Snickerdoodle Smoothie (p. 78)
Tropical Fruit Salad (p. 80)

Appetizers and Snacks

Almond Butter Bites (p. 82)
Gimme More Granola (p. 89)
Salsa (p. 96)
Spinach-Artichoke Dip (p. 97)
Tortilla Chips (p. 100)

Vegetables

Baked Potato Chips (p. 139)
Classic Tomato Sauce (p. 140)
Marinated Zucchini (p. 150)
Pan-Roasted Broccoli and Cauliflower (p. 152)

Salads, Soups, and Main Dishes

Butternut Squash and Broccoli Salad (p. 103)
Spinach Salad (p. 110)
Rice, Bean, and Sweet Potato Soup (p. 128)
Taco Soup (p. 130)
Chipotle Black Bean Burgers (p. 163)
Flatbread Pizza with Macadamia Nut Cheese (p. 166)
Lentil-Spinach "Meatballs" (p. 171)

Preparation Tips

- **Tropical Fruit Salad:** Can also be used for a quick snack.
- **Tortilla Chips:** Mix dough in the morning and store in refrigerator, covered in plastic wrap until ready to bake for dinner.
- **Classic Tomato Sauce:** Use with Pan-Roasted Broccoli and Cauliflower, Flatbread Pizza with Macadamia Nut Cheese, and Lentil-Spinach "Meatballs."
- **Rice, Bean, and Sweet Potato Soup:** Cook rice ahead of time and store in refrigerator.
- **Flatbread Pizza with Macadamia Nut Cheese:** Combine dough ingredients and store in refrigerator, covered with plastic wrap up to twenty-four hours before assembling pizza. Prepare Spinach-Artichoke Dip and Classic Tomato Sauce the night before you plan to make pizza.
- **Lentil-Spinach "Meatballs":** Cook lentils ahead of time.

Week 2 Combinations to Try

Tropical Fruit Salad with Gimme More Granola

Tortilla Chips with Salsa or Spinach-Artichoke Dip

Chipotle Black Bean Burgers with Baked Potato Chips

Flatbread Pizza with Macadamia Nut Cheese with Spinach Salad

Lentil-Spinach "Meatballs" with Classic Tomato Sauce

Week 3 Suggested Meal Plan

For a quick look at the ingredients for all of the recipes in this suggested meal plan, see pages 213–17.

Breakfast

Cinnamon Baked Apples (p. 73)
Fall Harvest Oatmeal (p. 75)
Fruit Pizza (p. 76)

Appetizers and Snacks

Corn Muffins (p. 86)
Green Salsa Bean Dip (p. 90)
Oatmeal Raisin Cookies (p. 93)
Pesto (p. 94)
Petite Pecan Pies (p. 94)

Vegetables

Ginger-Garlic Baby Carrots (p. 144)
Mashed Potato and Corn Casserole (p. 151)
Green Beans with Toasted Walnuts (p. 146)
Pesto Spaghetti Squash (p. 152)

Salads, Soups, and Main Dishes

Mediterranean Black Bean Salad (p. 105)
Ozarks Sunset Fruit Salad (p. 107)
Jamaican Chili (p. 126)
Vegetable Bean Soup (p. 133)
Caribbean Wild Rice (p. 162)
Greek-Style Stuffed Peppers (p. 168)
Spinach-Zucchini Casserole (p. 181)

Preparation Tips

- **Pesto Spaghetti Squash:** Make Pesto the day before.
- **Cinnamon Baked Apples:** Use in Fall Harvest Oatmeal.
- **Fruit Pizza:** Prepare dough and refrigerate, covered with plastic wrap until ready to assemble.
- **Corn Muffins:** Prepare dough and refrigerate, covered with plastic wrap until ready to bake.
- **Pesto:** Use to make Pesto Spaghetti Squash. Prepare Pesto one day ahead of time so flavors can blend.
- **Caribbean Wild Rice:** Chop vegetables in the morning and refrigerate in an airtight container until ready to cook at dinner.
- **Spinach-Zucchini Casserole:** Prepare the night before or in the morning. Make but don't bake, and store in refrigerator until ready to cook.

Week 3 Combinations to Try

Fall Harvest Oatmeal **with** Cinnamon Baked Apples

Mediterranean Black Bean Salad **with** Mashed Potato and Corn Casserole

Jamaican Chili **with** Corn Muffins

Vegetable Bean Soup **with** Ozarks Sunset Fruit Salad

Spinach-Zucchini Casserole **and** Green Beans with Toasted Walnuts

Breakfast Dishes

Apricot-Nut Breakfast Bar

YIELD: 12 servings
SERVING SIZE: 1 bar

1½ cups old-fashioned rolled oats

2 tablespoons flaxseed meal

½ cup unsweetened apple juice

1 tablespoon extra-virgin olive oil

¼ cup almond butter

¼ cup Date Honey (p. 87)

½ cup diced dried apricots (unsulfured)

¼ cup chopped macadamia nuts

2 tablespoons raw sunflower seeds

Preheat oven to 350 degrees. Toast oats in a large skillet over medium heat 5 – 7 minutes or until oats are golden, stirring frequently. Transfer to a large bowl, and add flaxseed meal, apple juice, olive oil, almond butter, and Date Honey. Mix until well combined. Stir in apricots, macadamia nuts, and sunflower seeds.

Press into an 8 by 8-inch square pan that has been lightly rubbed with olive oil. Bake 15 – 20 minutes. Let cool in pan on a wire rack about 5 minutes. Cut into 2 by 2½-inch bars and serve.

Recipe Notes
- Store in an airtight container 3 – 4 days.
- Substitute your favorite dried fruit for the apricots. Make sure, though, that the fruit doesn't contain any added sugar or preservatives.

Compounds containing sulfur are often added to dried foods as preservatives to help prevent oxidation and bleaching of colors. Instead of the bright-orange color of dried apricots treated with sulfite, unsulfured dried apricots are brown and are a much healthier choice.

Baked Oatmeal

1½ cups old-fashioned rolled oats

1½ cups unsweetened almond milk

½ cup unsweetened applesauce

¼ cup chopped dried apricots

¼ cup chopped dates or raisins

¼ cup chopped pecans or walnuts

½ teaspoon cinnamon

¼ teaspoon salt

YIELD: 6 servings
SERVING SIZE:
  2 squares

Preheat oven to 350 degrees. Put all ingredients in a large bowl and stir well. Transfer to an 8 by 8-inch baking dish that has been lightly rubbed with olive oil. Pour oatmeal mixture into dish and bake 45–50 minutes or until slightly browned and crispy on top.

Recipe Notes

- Spread almond butter or Date Honey on each serving.
- Top with Cinnamon Baked Apples.
- Makes a great afternoon snack.
- This recipe can be doubled and baked in a 9 by 13-inch casserole dish.

Old-fashioned oats are oat groats that have been steamed and run through rollers to flatten them out. They have a mild, slightly nutty flavor and tend to be chewier than quick oats, which have been flaked to cook more quickly. Old-fashioned oats are a whole grain, since they contain the nutrient-rich germ and the bran, which is extremely high in fiber.

Banana-Fig Oatmeal with Almond Butter

⅔ cup old-fashioned rolled oats

1 tablespoon almond butter

1 tablespoon flaxseed meal

1 banana, peeled and sliced (about 1 cup)

¼ cup diced dried figs

1 tablespoon finely chopped walnuts

¼ teaspoon cinnamon

YIELD: 2 servings
SERVING SIZE:
  about ¾ cup

Cook oats on stovetop according to package directions. Stir in almond butter and flaxseed meal until well combined. Add banana slices, figs, walnuts, and cinnamon.

Recipe Notes
- Add 1 tablespoon Date Honey to each serving.
- Use raisins instead of dried figs.
- Substitute ½ cup dry steel-cut oats for the rolled oats. Steel-cut oats are whole grain groats (the inner portion of the oat kernel) which have been cut into only two or three pieces by steel rather than being rolled. They are golden in color and resemble small rice pieces. This form of oats takes longer to prepare than rolled oats (typically 15 – 30 minutes to simmer). Cooked steel-cut oats are chewier and taste nuttier than regular oats.

> Flaxseed meal is a powder made from ground flaxseeds. It is high in fiber and a good source of omega-3 fatty acids. It can be found in health food stores and some grocery stores. Instead of buying flaxseed meal, you can also grind whole flaxseeds at home by using a coffee or seed grinder.

Broiled Pineapple Slices

YIELD: 6 servings
SERVING SIZE: 1 slice

6 fresh or canned pineapple slices
1 tablespoon Date Honey (p. 87)
1 tablespoon fresh lime juice
1 tablespoon unsweetened coconut flakes

Turn oven to broil setting. Place pineapple slices on a broiler pan lined with foil or on an 11 by 17-inch baking sheet rubbed with olive oil. Mix Date Honey and lime juice in a small bowl. Spread on top side of pineapple. Place 3 – 4 inches below broiler for about 8 minutes. Remove from oven and sprinkle each slice with ½ teaspoon coconut flakes. Broil for 2 minutes and serve.

Recipe Notes
- Cut slices into chunks and mix in with oatmeal. Add chopped dates or raisins.

- Omit the coconut flakes and just spread Date Honey and lime juice on top.

When selecting pineapple, choose one that is plump and looks fresh. The leaves in the crown should be green, and the body of the pineapple firm. Avoid pineapples that have soft spots or visible damage. The larger the pineapple, the greater the proportion of edible fruit. However, a larger pineapple doesn't necessarily taste sweeter than a smaller one.

Cinnamon Baked Apples

2 cups thinly sliced apples, unpeeled (about 2 apples)
1 cup unsweetened apple juice
⅛ teaspoon cinnamon

YIELD: 4 servings
SERVING SIZE:
   about ½ cup

Preheat oven to 350 degrees. Place sliced apples in an 8 by 8-inch baking dish. In a small bowl, whisk apple juice and cinnamon, and pour over apples. Bake 15 minutes, stir, and bake another 15 minutes. Serve warm.

Recipe Notes
- Serve with oatmeal or cooked brown rice.
- Pour over Baked Oatmeal.
- Sprinkle unsweetened coconut flakes and/or chopped pecans on top.
- Add sliced bananas, raisins, and chopped nuts.
- Substitute pears for the apples.

The best baking apples are ones that are firm, with a good balance of sweetness and tartness, and with flesh that won't break down as it cooks. A few of the types that are recommended are:

- *Golden Delicious:* sweet with a crisp, juicy texture; one of the best varieties for baking.
- *Granny Smith:* mildly tart green apples.
- *Gala:* yellow-orange skin with red striping and with a creamy yellow flesh inside; mild and sweet.
- *Jonathan:* red and green with a crunchy texture and a sweet-tart flavor.
- *Rome:* red with a light green flesh; crisp and mildly tart.

Coconut Fig Bars

YIELD: 12 servings
SERVING SIZE: 1 bar

½ cup coconut flour
½ cup old-fashioned rolled oats
1 cup unsweetened applesauce
¼ cup Date Honey (p. 87)
1 cup chopped dried figs
2 tablespoons chopped pecans
1 tablespoon flaxseed meal (optional)
1 tablespoon unsweetened shredded coconut
½ teaspoon cinnamon

Preheat oven to 350 degrees. In a large bowl, mix coconut flour, oats, applesauce, and Date Honey until well combined. Stir in figs, pecans, flaxseed meal (optional), coconut, and cinnamon.

Lightly rub an 8 by 8-inch baking dish with olive oil and press mixture into dish. Bake 15 minutes or until top is lightly browned. Cool 10 minutes at room temperature and serve.

Recipe Notes
- Substitute almond flour, oat flour, or whole wheat flour for coconut flour. Increase shredded coconut to ¼ cup to maintain the coconut flavor.
- Spread ½ tablespoon of almond butter or Date Honey on top of each serving.
- Instead of buying flaxseed meal, you can also grind whole flaxseeds at home using a coffee or seed grinder.

Coconut flour is made from fresh coconut meat that has been finely ground into a powder with most of the moisture and fat removed. It is a delicious, healthy alternative to wheat and other grain flours. Coconut flour is also very high in fiber, a good source of protein, and gluten-free. You can find coconut flour at most health food stores or purchase it online.

Fall Harvest Oatmeal

½ recipe Cinnamon Baked Apples (p. 73)

⅔ cup old-fashioned rolled oats

4 Medjool dates, pitted, chopped (about ¼ cup)

2 tablespoons chopped pecans

¼ cup apple juice (from Cinnamon Baked Apples recipe)

Prepare Cinnamon Baked Apples as directed. When apples are done, cook oats on stovetop according to package directions. To serve, place ½ cup oatmeal in two bowls. Top with apples, dates, and pecans. Pour 2 tablespoons of apple juice over each serving, and serve immediately.

Recipe Notes

- Use figs or raisins instead of dates.
- Substitute pears for apples.
- Since you need only half of the Cinnamon Baked Apples recipe, you can store the other half in an airtight container in the refrigerator and use the following day.
- Substitute ½ cup dry steel-cut oats for the rolled oats. Steel-cut oats are whole grain groats (the inner portion of the oat kernel) which have been cut into only two or three pieces by steel rather than being rolled. They are golden in color and resemble small rice pieces. This form of oats takes longer to prepare than rolled oats (typically 15 – 30 minutes to simmer). Cooked steel-cut oats are chewier and taste nuttier than regular oats.

To keep pecans fresh and flavorful, you must store them properly. Because pecans have a high oil content, they are more likely than most other nuts to become rancid at warm temperatures. Airtight containers, such as jars with tight-fitting lids, are best for storing pecans in the refrigerator. Sealed plastic bags are best for the freezer.

Breakfast Dishes

Fruit Pizza

YIELD: 8 servings
SERVING SIZE: 1 slice

Crust

1½ cups almond flour (meal)

½ cup roughly chopped pitted dates

½ cup chopped pecans

¼ cup unsweetened apple juice

Fruit Sauce

¼ cup Date Honey (p. 87)

½ cup sliced strawberries

Topping Ideas

Sliced apples, bananas, blueberries, grapes, kiwifruit, mangoes, oranges, peaches, pineapples, strawberries

Preheat oven to 350 degrees. Place almond flour, dates, pecans, and apple juice in a food processor. Process until mixture forms a ball. Press dough into a 10-inch circle, about ¼-inch thick, on an 11 by 17-inch baking sheet or pizza pan. (Rub a little olive oil on your hands if dough gets too sticky.) With a fork, poke holes all across crust dough. Bake 10 minutes, or until edges are browned and slightly crispy. Remove from oven and let cool completely, about 45 minutes.

Put Date Honey and strawberries in a food processor or blender. Process about 30 seconds or until smooth and creamy. Spread fruit sauce onto cooled crust. Top with your favorite assortment of sliced fruit. Refrigerate 3 hours or until chilled.

Recipe Notes
- Top with toasted unsweetened shredded coconut flakes.
- Use ½ cup blueberries in the fruit sauce instead of strawberries.
- Add 2 ounces silken tofu and ¼ teaspoon cinnamon for a creamier fruit sauce.
- Substitute oat flour for the almond flour.
- Serve with only the fruit sauce as a topping.

> Another great way to enjoy Fruit Pizza is to put it in the freezer to cool for 30–45 minutes to make a tasty, frozen dessert.

Nutty Fruit Cereal

1   banana, peeled and sliced (about 1 cup)
⅓   cup fresh blueberries
1   tablespoon chopped almonds
1   tablespoon chopped walnuts
1   teaspoon unsweetened coconut flakes
½   cup unsweetened almond or rice milk

YIELD: 1 serving
SERVING SIZE:
   about 1⅓ cups

Place banana slices in a bowl and top with blueberries, almonds, walnuts, and coconut flakes. Pour in almond milk.

Recipe Notes

• Add ½ tablespoon sunflower seeds.
• Substitute chopped pecans for the almonds or walnuts.
• Enjoy as a fruit and nut snack without the almond milk.
• Other fruit ideas are apples, blackberries, kiwifruit, peaches, pears, or strawberries.

Blueberries may be little, but they have a big nutritional profile. They are often considered a "superfood" because of their high level of disease-fighting antioxidants.

Pineapple Citrus Muffins

1   cup old-fashioned rolled oats
1   cup oat flour (see Recipe Notes)
1   cup unsweetened applesauce
½   cup diced pineapple
¼   cup chopped pecans or walnuts
¼   cup Date Honey (p. 87)
¼   cup flaxseed meal
2   teaspoons unsweetened coconut flakes
2   teaspoons grated orange zest
½   teaspoon ground ginger

YIELD: 8 servings
SERVING SIZE: 1 muffin

Preheat oven to 350 degrees. Lightly rub 8 cups of a 12-cup muffin tin with olive oil, and set aside.

Combine all ingredients in a large bowl, and stir well to combine. Scoop out mixture into muffin tin cups, allowing about ⅓ cup for each muffin. Bake 20 minutes, or until muffin tops are lightly browned. Serve warm.

Recipe Notes

- Make your own oat flour by placing old-fashioned rolled oats in a food processor or blender and process until fine (1 cup old-fashioned oats will yield about ¾ cup ground oats).
- Spread almond butter or Date Honey on top.
- Flaxseed meal is a powder made from ground flaxseeds. It can be found in health food stores and some grocery stores. Instead of buying flaxseed meal, you can also grind whole flaxseeds at home using a coffee or seed grinder.
- The zest is the outermost, colorful skin of citrus fruits. Zest is often used to enhance flavor in recipes. The pith, or white membrane underneath the outside peel, has a bitter, unpleasant taste and should be avoided while zesting.

Pineapples are high in vitamin C and can help strengthen your immune system to fight against colds and the flu. They also contain bromelain, an enzyme which has been known to soothe symptoms of sinusitis.

Snickerdoodle Smoothie

YIELD: 2 servings
SERVING SIZE: about 1½ cups

6 ounces silken tofu
½ cup unsweetened almond or rice milk
¼ cup Date Honey (p. 87)
2 frozen bananas, peeled, sliced (about 2 cups)
1 teaspoon cinnamon
⅛ teaspoon nutmeg

Place tofu, almond milk, Date Honey, banana slices, cinnamon, and nutmeg in blender. Mix until smooth.

Recipe Notes

- Remove peels before placing bananas in freezer. Put in a plastic zip-top bag until completely frozen.

- Instead of using Date Honey, soak 3 – 4 Medjool dates in warm water at room temperature for an hour before adding to blender.
- Add flaxseed meal for extra fiber.
- You can also use firm tofu for this recipe. However, you may want to add more almond milk if the consistency is too thick.

Instead of drinking your smoothie, make popsicles with it. Pour the blended smoothie into popsicle molds, and put it in the freezer overnight. The next day, you can enjoy a creamy, refreshing Snickerdoodle Smoothie treat!

Strawberry-Banana Smoothie

4 ounces extra-firm tofu

¼ cup unsweetened almond milk

¼ cup unsweetened apple juice

2 tablespoons Date Honey (p. 87)

1 cup sliced strawberries

1 frozen banana, peeled, sliced (about 1 cup)

YIELD: 2 servings
SERVING SIZE:
about 1 cup

Place all ingredients in a blender, and process until smooth.

Recipe Notes

- Remove peels before placing bananas in freezer. Put in a plastic zip-top bag until completely frozen.
- Add flaxseed meal for extra fiber.
- Instead of using Date Honey, soak 3 – 4 Medjool dates in warm water at room temperature for an hour before adding to blender.
- Substitute 1 cup chopped kiwifruit for bananas.

Bananas are an exceptionally rich source of fructo-oligosaccharide, a compound that nourishes probiotic (friendly) bacteria in the colon. These beneficial bacteria produce enzymes that increase our digestive ability and protect us from unhealthy bacterial infections.

Tropical Fruit Salad

YIELD: 6 servings
SERVING SIZE:
about 1 cup

2 cups sliced strawberries

3 kiwifruit, peeled and quartered

1½ cups orange segments, cut into 1-inch pieces

1 cup red seedless grapes, halved

1 cup fresh pineapple chunks, diced

Mix fruit in a large bowl, and chill until ready to serve.

Recipe Notes

- Use mandarin oranges instead of regular oranges.
- Top with chopped almonds, macadamia nuts, pecans, and/or walnuts.
- Sprinkle lightly toasted unsweetened shredded coconut on top.
- Other fruit choices are apples, bananas, blueberries, peaches, and/or mangoes. However, if you do use apples or bananas, mix in a little lemon juice with fruit to prevent browning.

Kiwifruit adds a tropical flair to this colorful fruit salad. It's a small fruit, usually only about three inches long, with a fuzzy, brown peel. Inside the kiwifruit is a bright green flesh with a white pulp in the center that's surrounded by black, edible seeds. Kiwifruit has a sweet taste, similar to a mixture of banana, pineapple, and strawberry. The greatest nutritional benefit the kiwifruit offers is that it is packed with vitamin C.

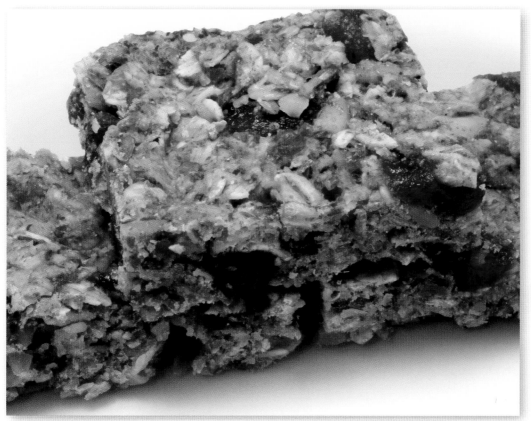

Apricot-Nut Breakfast Bar (p. 70)

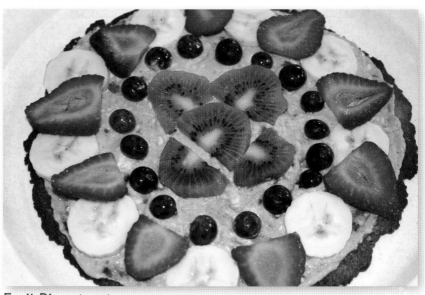

Fruit Pizza (p. 76)

Breakfast Dishes

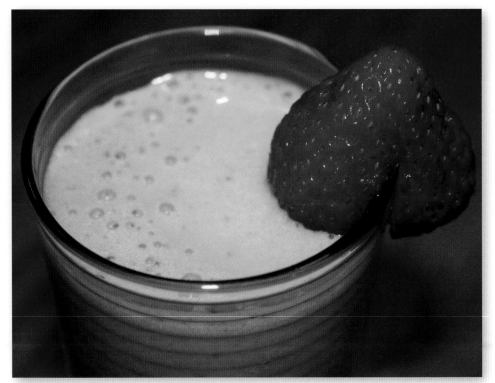

Strawberry-Banana Smoothie (p. 79)

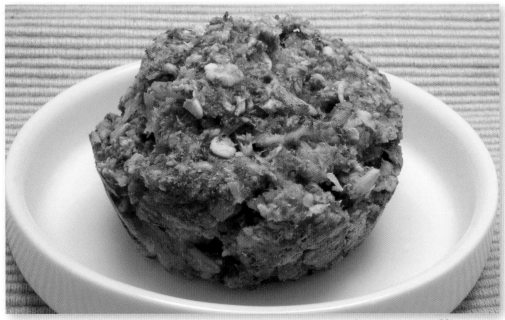

Pineapple Citrus Muffin (p. 77)

Appetizers and Snacks

Appetizers and Snacks

Almond Butter Bites

½ cup almond butter

¼ cup raw sunflower seeds

¼ cup raisins

¼ cup chopped almonds

2 tablespoons unsweetened shredded coconut

¼ teaspoon cinnamon

Mix all ingredients in a bowl until well combined. Use a ½ tablespoon measuring spoon or a large melon ball scoop to form mixture into small balls. Place in an 8 by 8-inch baking dish, and freeze 2 – 3 hours or until firm. Serve frozen or just slightly thawed.

Recipe Notes
• Substitute chopped dried apricots, figs, or dates for the raisins.

Almond butter is a tasty alternative to peanut butter. Although it is somewhat expensive, its naturally sweet taste will win you over. Almonds are high in protein, fiber, and calcium. They're also an excellent source of monounsaturated fats — the heart-healthy type that helps to lower cholesterol and reduce the risk of heart disease.

Black Bean Dip

1 tablespoon extra-virgin olive oil

1 cup diced onion

1 cup diced red bell peppers (about 1 large pepper)

1 clove garlic, minced

½ cup water

2 (15-ounce) cans black beans, rinsed and drained

2 tablespoons fresh parsley or 1½ teaspoons dried parsley

½ teaspoon dried crushed rosemary

¼ teaspoon salt

⅛ teaspoon pepper

Heat olive oil in a large skillet over medium heat. Add onions and red peppers, and cook until onions are soft and translucent. Stir in garlic, and cook for 30 seconds, stirring constantly so garlic doesn't burn.

Place water and 2 cups of beans in food processor or blender; process until smooth. Pour the pureed beans into skillet and stir. Add the remaining beans, parsley, rosemary, salt, and pepper. Reduce heat to low and cook 15 minutes, stirring occasionally. Transfer to a serving dish and serve warm.

Recipe Notes

- Serve with Tortilla Chips.
- Use as a topping for baked potatoes.
- Spread on top of Broiled Polenta Squares or Corn Muffins.
- Add ¼ cup Salsa.

Black beans, or turtle beans, are practically a staple for anyone doing the Daniel Fast. When cooked, black beans have a rich, almost meaty taste. Combine them with a whole grain, such as brown rice or quinoa, and you have a high quality protein dish. Black beans are also low on the glycemic index, which means that your blood sugar level doesn't rise too rapidly after eating them, which is especially beneficial for individuals with diabetes, insulin resistance, or hypoglycemia.

Broiled Polenta Squares

6 cups water

1 tablespoon salt

2½ cups yellow cornmeal

1 teaspoon dried basil or oregano

½ teaspoon garlic powder

YIELD: 9 servings
SERVING SIZE:
  2 squares (2½ inches)

Heat water to boiling in a large saucepan. Add salt. Reduce heat to bring water to a simmer; slowly pour cornmeal in a thin stream into the saucepan. Stir constantly with a whisk to prevent clumping. After adding all the cornmeal, stir with a wooden spoon until the polenta is thick and pulls away from the sides of the pan; this may take 15 – 20 minutes. For best results, stir constantly until the polenta has reached this consistency.

Wet a paper towel, and rub the bottom and sides of a 9 by 13-inch casserole dish with water to prevent sticking. Once polenta has cooked, transfer it to the dish. With a rubber spatula, press polenta until it is well packed. Cover with plastic wrap and refrigerate 2 hours or until completely cooled.

Preheat oven to broil setting. Using a paper towel, rub a large 11 by 17-inch baking sheet with olive oil and set aside. Remove casserole dish from refrigerator and cut polenta into 2½-inch squares. Place squares on prepared baking sheet, and place 3 – 4 inches under broiler. Bake 15 minutes, flip, and bake 15 minutes more. Both sides should be crispy before serving.

Recipe Notes
- Top squares with a dollop of Black Bean Dip, Confetti Hummus, Hummus, Guacamole with a Little Kick, or Spinach-Artichoke Dip.
- Pour Artichoke Tomato Sauce or Eggplant Tomato Sauce over squares.
- Serve with Black Bean Chili Bake or Mexican Rice and Beans.
- Goes well with Black Bean Minestrone, Taco Soup, or Tuscan Soup.
- Store half of the broiled squares in an airtight container in the freezer for later use.

> Polenta is a popular food in Italian cooking. It's made from ground cornmeal, which is then boiled in water to create a porridge-like substance. Enjoy polenta right off the stove while it's hot or bake it for a crispier texture.

Cinnamon Roasted Almonds

    2 cups whole almonds
    ½ tablespoon extra-virgin olive oil
    ½ teaspoon cinnamon
    ¼ teaspoon salt

YIELD: 8 servings
SERVING SIZE:
  about ¼ cup

Preheat oven to 250 degrees. Line an 11 by 17-inch baking sheet with parchment paper or lightly rub with olive oil and set aside. Put almonds in a large bowl, add olive oil, and stir well. Sprinkle in cinnamon and salt and toss to coat.

Spread almonds evenly on baking sheet. Bake 1 hour, stirring occasionally. Cool and serve, or store in an airtight container.

Recipe Notes
• Chop almonds and serve with oatmeal.
• Sprinkle on top of chopped apples or sliced bananas for a healthy snack.
• Add ¼ teaspoon cumin.
• Instead of cinnamon, use chipotle chili pepper seasoning, chili powder, or Taco Seasoning to make spicy flavored almonds.

Keep almonds in a cool dry place away from exposure to sunlight to prolong their freshness. Refrigerated almonds will keep for several months. Almonds stored in the freezer can be kept up to a year.

Confetti Hummus

    1 (15-ounce) can chickpeas, rinsed and drained
    ½ cup chopped canned artichokes, drained
    ½ chopped jarred roasted red bell peppers, drained
    ¼ cup tahini
    ¼ cup water
    2 tablespoons extra-virgin olive oil
    2 tablespoons fresh lemon juice
    2 cloves garlic, minced
    ¼ cup fresh parsley, packed

YIELD: 10 servings
SERVING SIZE:
  about ¼ cup

½ teaspoon salt

¼ teaspoon ground cumin

Place all ingredients in a food processor or blender. Process, scraping sides of bowl often, until mixture is a smooth paste. Refrigerate, or serve immediately.

Recipe Notes

• Serve as a dip for fresh vegetables.
• Use as a filling for Romaine Wraps or Whole Grain Tortillas.
• Spread on top of fresh tomato slices.
• Use as the main ingredient in Hummus Casserole.
• Tahini is a thick paste made from ground sesame seeds. It is a staple in Middle Eastern cooking and can be found at health food stores and most large grocery-store chains.

Chickpeas, or garbanzo beans, provide a high amount of fiber and can help lower cholesterol. They can also help to improve blood sugar levels, which makes them a healthy choice for people who have diabetes or are insulin resistant.

Corn Muffins

YIELD: 12 servings
SERVING SIZE:
2 mini muffins or
1 regular muffin

1½ cups yellow cornmeal

½ cup unsweetened almond or rice milk

¼ cup water

1 tablespoon Date Honey (p. 87) (optional)

1 tablespoon extra-virgin olive oil

¾ cup fresh or frozen corn kernels

¼ cup chopped green onions (green parts only)

½ teaspoon salt

Preheat oven to 400 degrees. Mix cornmeal, almond milk, water, Date Honey, and olive oil in a medium bowl. Stir until well combined. Add corn, green onions, and salt. Mix well.

Lightly rub a mini-muffin tin with olive oil. Fill all 24 cups about ¾ full and bake 15 minues. If using a regular muffin tin, fill all 12 cups about ¾ full and bake 20 minutes.

Recipe Notes

- Use 1½ tablespoons dried chives instead of green onions.
- Serve with Black-and-White Chili, Jamaican Chili, Tuscan Soup, or Vegetable Bean Soup.

> Cornmeal is flour ground from dried corn. It is sometimes referred to as corn flour.

Date Honey

1 cup pitted dates (about 6 – 8 Medjool or 18 – 20 Deglet Noor)
1 cup water
½ teaspoon cinnamon

YIELD: 12 servings
SERVING SIZE:
about 1 tablespoon

Pour dates and water into a small saucepan, making sure dates are completely covered. (Add additional water if necessary.) Bring to a boil over high heat. Reduce heat to low and simmer 45 – 60 minutes or until dates are very soft and broken down. Remove from heat, and allow to cool slightly for about 15 minutes. Pour mixture into a blender or food processor and puree until smooth. Sprinkle in cinnamon and stir well. Store in a sealed container in refrigerator.

Recipe Notes

- Serve with sliced apples, pears, and/or bananas.
- Use to make Coconut Fig Bars, Fruit Pizza, Oatmeal Raisin Cookies, Pineapple Citrus Muffins, and Snickerdoodle Smoothie, Strawberry-Banana Smoothie, and Sweet Potato Pie.
- Spread on top of a slice of Baked Oatmeal.

> Dates are high in natural sugars, making them an ideal energy-boosting snack.

Appetizers and Snacks

Flatbread

YIELD: 4 servings
SERVING SIZE: 2 pieces

2½ cups whole grain flour (brown rice, spelt, whole wheat, etc.)
2 tablespoons flaxseed meal (optional)
1 teaspoon dried crushed rosemary
1 teaspoon salt
1 cup warm water
1 tablespoon extra-virgin olive oil
½ teaspoon dried basil
½ teaspoon garlic powder
½ teaspoon dried parsley

Mix flour, flaxseed meal, rosemary, salt, and water in a food processor until dough forms a ball. Turn dough onto a floured work surface, and knead for 5 minutes. Transfer to a bowl, and cover tightly with plastic wrap. Let dough rest at room temperature 30–60 minutes.

Preheat oven to 400 degrees. Roll dough out to ¼-inch thickness to cover an oiled 11 by 17-inch baking sheet. With a fork, poke holes all across dough. Mix olive oil, basil, garlic powder, and parsley in a small bowl, and stir well. Use a basting brush to spread oil mixture across dough. Score (make shallow cuts without separating into pieces) with a knife into 12 (3 by 3½-inch) squares. Bake 15–20 minutes or until slightly crispy, and remove from oven. Let cool on baking sheet 10 minutes before cutting and serving.

Recipe Notes
• Make this a sweet-tasting flatbread by using ½ teaspoon cinnamon instead of basil, garlic powder, and parsley.
• Flaxseed meal is a powder made from ground flaxseeds. It can be found in health food stores and some grocery stores. Instead of buying flaxseed meal, you can also grind whole flaxseeds at home using a coffee or seed grinder.

A flatbread is a simple bread made with flour, water, and salt and then thoroughly rolled into flattened dough. Many flatbreads, such as the one in this recipe, are unleavened, or made without yeast.

Gimme More Granola

¼ cup chopped dried plums (prunes) or pitted dates

¼ cup water

1 cup old-fashioned rolled oats

2 tablespoons unsweetened apple juice

1 tablespoon extra-virgin olive oil

¼ cup raisins

2 tablespoons chopped almonds

2 tablespoons chopped walnuts

2 tablespoons raw sunflower seeds

2 tablespoons unsweetened shredded coconut

YIELD: 8 servings
SERVING SIZE:
about ¼ cup

Preheat oven to 350 degrees. In a small saucepan, add plums and water. Cook over medium heat 5 minutes or until plums are softened. Transfer to a food processor or blender and process until mixture is a thick paste, about 30 seconds.

In a large bowl, combine plum mixture, oats, apple juice, olive oil, raisins, almonds, walnuts, sunflower seeds, and coconut. Stir until well combined.

Spread mixture into an even layer on an 11 by 17-inch baking sheet that has been lined with parchment paper or lightly rubbed with olive oil. Bake 5 minutes, stir, and bake another 5 minutes, or until lightly browned. Let cool on pan. Granola will become crispy as it cools. Store in an airtight container at room temperature for about 2 weeks or up to 1 month in the refrigerator.

Recipe Notes
- Substitute pecans or cashews for almonds and walnuts.
- Serve with fresh fruit and almond milk for breakfast.
- Use chopped dried apricots instead of raisins.
- Add raw pumpkin seeds (pepitas).

Granola is truly the perfect healthy snack. It's easy to make and packed with fiber, protein, vitamins, and minerals. Granola is also very filling and satisfying—a little goes a long way.

Great Northern Dip

YIELD: 8 servings
SERVING SIZE:
about 2 tablespoons

1 (15-ounce) can great northern beans, rinsed and drained
2 tablespoons water
¼ cup green onions (green parts only), chopped coarse
1 clove garlic, minced
1 tablespoon chopped fresh oregano or 1 teaspoon dried oregano flakes
¼ teaspoon salt

Place all ingredients in a food processor or blender and puree until smooth.

Recipe Notes
• Serve with fresh vegetables.
• Spread on top of tomato slices.
• Use as a filling for Romaine Wraps or Whole Grain Tortillas.
• Use as a dip with Tortilla Chips.

> Great northern beans are mildly flavored white beans that readily take on the flavor of spices or herbs used in cooking. Any recipe that uses other white beans, such as navy beans or cannellini beans, can be made with great northern beans.

Green Salsa Bean Dip

YIELD: 16 servings
SERVING SIZE:
about 2 tablespoons

1 (15-ounce) can great northern beans, rinsed and drained
1 (10-ounce) can diced tomatoes and green chilies, undrained
2 cups chopped kale or spinach, lightly packed
2 cloves garlic, minced
½ teaspoon salt

Place all ingredients in a food processor or blender. Process until smooth.

Recipe Notes
• Serve with fresh vegetables.
• Use as a dip with Tortilla Chips.
• Stir a couple of tablespoons into your salad instead of using an oil-based dressing.

- Kale is a leafy green vegetable with a fibrous stalk and ruffled leaves. To prepare kale, remove and discard tough stems and use only the leaves.

One night my husband asked me to make a fresh batch of Salsa. I didn't have all of the necessary ingredients on hand, so I rummaged through my pantry to see what I could come up with. The result was Green Salsa Bean Dip, which was a pleasant surprise for both of us! I couldn't believe that just a few ingredients could make such a tasty salsa-flavored dip. My husband liked it so much that as soon as the dip was gone, he asked me to make it again. That's always a good sign.

Guacamole with a Little Kick

2 medium avocados
½ cup chopped tomatoes, unpeeled, unseeded
¼ cup diced red onion
½ medium jalapeno pepper, seeded and diced
1 clove garlic, minced
2 tablespoons chopped fresh parsley or cilantro
1 tablespoon fresh lime juice
½ teaspoon salt

YIELD: 6 servings
SERVING SIZE:
  about ¼ cup

Cut avocados in half and remove the seeds. Use a large spoon to scoop out the flesh. Put in a small mixing bowl, and mash with a fork until smooth. Stir in the rest of the ingredients. Mix well. Chill 1 – 2 hours before serving.

Recipe Notes
- For even more kick, use the whole jalapeno. Also, keeping the seeds in the dip will add more heat.
- Add ½ cup Salsa.

The trick to perfect guacamole is using good, ripe avocados. Check for ripeness by gently pressing the outside of the avocado. If there is no give, the avocado is not ready. If there is a lot of give, the avocado is ripe. Beware of too much softness, though, because usually that means the avocado may be too ripe and won't taste good.

Another test is to flick off the small stem on the avocado. If it comes off easily, the avocado is ripe. If it doesn't come off, the avocado shouldn't be eaten yet.

Hummus

1 (15-ounce) can chickpeas, rinsed and drained
¼ cup tahini
¼ cup water
2 tablespoons extra-virgin olive oil
2 tablespoons fresh lemon juice
2 cloves garlic, minced
¼ cup fresh parsley, packed
½ teaspoon salt
¼ teaspoon ground cumin

Place all ingredients in a food processor or blender. Process until mixture is a smooth paste, scraping down the sides of the bowl several times. Refrigerate or serve immediately.

Recipe Notes

• Use as a dip for fresh vegetables, such as bell peppers, broccoli, carrots, celery, cucumber slices, black olives, sugar snap peas, and zucchini slices.
• Substitute black beans for the chickpeas or use ½ can of each.
• Spread on fresh tomato slices.
• Stir a couple of tablespoons into your salad instead of using an oil-based dressing.
• Use as the main ingredient in Hummus Casserole.
• Add roasted red bell peppers and artichokes to make Confetti Hummus.

Hummus tastes best when refrigerated twenty-four hours before serving, which allows flavors to blend. It can be refrigerated up to a week and frozen up to three months.

Oatmeal Raisin Cookies

1 cup old-fashioned rolled oats

1 cup almond flour or oat flour (see Recipe Notes)

1 cup creamy cashew butter, almond butter, or peanut butter

½ cup unsweetened applesauce

⅓ cup Date Honey (p. 87)

½ cup raisins

2 tablespoons chopped walnuts

1 teaspoon cinnamon

YIELD: 18 – 20 servings
SERVING SIZE: 1 cookie

Preheat oven to 350 degrees. Mix oats, almond flour, cashew butter, applesauce, and Date Honey in a large bowl until well combined. Add raisins, walnuts, and cinnamon. Stir well.

Drop by spoonfuls, two inches apart, on an 11 by 17-inch baking sheet. Flatten and shape into circles. Bake 10 – 12 minutes.

Recipe Notes

• Make your own oat flour by placing old-fashioned rolled oats in a food processor or blender and process until fine (1 cup old-fashioned oats will yield about ¾ cup ground oats).

• Increase the applesauce to 1 cup if you don't use Date Honey.

• Instead of using 1 cup almond flour, use ½ cup old-fashioned rolled oats and ½ cup almond or oat flour.

Raisins are high in iron, the nutrient responsible for the formation of hemoglobin, which carries oxygen to all body cells. Iron also aids in immune function, cognitive development, temperature regulation, and energy metabolism.

Appetizers and Snacks

Pesto

YIELD: 6 servings
SERVING SIZE:
about 2 tablespoons

2 tablespoons extra-virgin olive oil

3 cups fresh spinach leaves, packed

¼ cup chopped green onions

¼ cup pine nuts or walnuts

2 cloves garlic, minced

½ cup packed fresh basil leaves

¼ teaspoon salt

Place ingredients in a food processor or blender until smooth. If pesto seems too thick, add a little hot water.

Recipe Notes

- Substitute ½ (10-ounce) package of frozen chopped spinach (thawed and squeezed dry) for fresh spinach leaves.
- Use as the main ingredient in Pesto Spaghetti Squash.
- Spread on fresh tomato slices.
- Serve with Tortilla Chips or Whole Grain Tortillas.
- Works great as a sauce for Flatbread Pizza with Macadamia Nut Cheese.

Basil, the star ingredient in pesto, is an aromatic herb originally from India (not Italy, as is sometimes assumed), and the most common variety is green with large, soft leaves.

Petite Pecan Pies

YIELD: 4 servings
SERVING SIZE: 2 pies

8 Medjool dates

8 pecan halves

Remove pits from dates. Stuff one pecan half into each date.

Recipe Notes

- Medjool dates are the largest variety of dates and work best with pecan halves.
- Stuff with almond butter instead of pecans.

Medjool dates could easily be described as nature's candy. Known as the "king of dates," they are exceptionally large and super sweet. The center of the date has an elongated pit. Once the pit is removed, you can eat the date or stuff it with nuts or nut butter. To store dates, put them in a tightly closed container in the freezer or refrigerator. When stored frozen, dates can retain their quality for up to one year.

Roasted Chickpeas

2 (15-ounce) cans chickpeas, rinsed and drained
1 tablespoon extra-virgin olive oil
½ teaspoon garlic powder
½ teaspoon onion powder
½ teaspoon dried crushed rosemary
¼ teaspoon salt

YIELD: 8 servings
SERVING SIZE:
about ¼ cup

Preheat oven to 350 degrees. Lightly rub an 11 by 17-inch baking sheet with olive oil. Spread chickpeas out in a single layer on the sheet.

Roast about 20 minutes, or until chickpeas are dry to the touch. Remove from oven, and increase temperature to 425 degrees. Place chickpeas in a large bowl. Add olive oil, garlic powder, onion powder, rosemary, and salt. Stir until well coated.

Return to baking sheet and roast another 15 – 20 minutes (double-roasting the chickpeas gives them a crunchy texture), or until the chickpeas are crispy and lightly browned. Let cool completely on baking sheet before serving or storing.

Recipe Notes
• Use as a salad topping.
• Make spicy chickpeas by using Taco Seasoning or chili powder instead of the garlic powder, onion powder, and rosemary.

Roasted chickpeas tend to lose their crispiness even when stored in an airtight container, so they're best when eaten immediately. However, if you do store them for a day or two, you might need to heat them in the oven a few minutes to dry them out and restore their crunch.

Salsa

YIELD: 12 servings
SERVING SIZE:
about ¼ cup

3 – 4 large tomatoes, unpeeled, unseeded, quartered
1 (10-ounce) can diced tomatoes and green chilies, undrained
½ cup chopped green bell peppers
½ cup chopped red bell peppers
½ cup chopped red onion
1 serrano pepper, seeded and chopped
¼ cup packed fresh cilantro or parsley
2 – 3 cloves garlic, minced
1 tablespoon fresh lime juice
½ teaspoon salt
¼ teaspoon cumin

Add all ingredients to a food processor or blender; pulse until desired consistency is reached. Chill at least 1 hour to let flavors blend.

Recipe Notes

• Use as a dip for fresh vegetables.
• Serve with Tortilla Chips.
• Mix in a salad instead of using an oil-based dressing.
• Works great as a topping for a baked potato or South of the Border Pizza.
• If you prefer a milder salsa, use ¼ teaspoon of crushed red pepper instead of the fresh serrano pepper. If you like your salsa super spicy, use a hotter pepper, such as a jalapeno.
• Use 1 (14.5-ounce) can undrained diced tomatoes instead of fresh tomatoes.

Fresh serrano chilies can be found in the produce section of most supermarkets. Choose peppers with a deep green color, avoiding chilies that appear wrinkled or feel soft. Store in a plastic bag for up to two weeks in the refrigerator.

The seeds and membranes contain most of the capsaicin, which is what gives them their mouth-searing qualities. Use caution when handling. Serranos are hot enough to irritate the skin on the hands, and it can be painful if their juice comes into contact with the eyes. Wear thin disposable gloves while working with them, and don't touch your face until the gloves are removed.

Spicy Pumpkin Seeds

2 teaspoons extra-virgin olive oil

1 teaspoon Taco Seasoning (p. 98) or chili powder

1 cup whole raw pumpkin seeds (pepitas)

YIELD: 4 servings
SERVING SIZE:
about ¼ cup

Preheat oven to 275 degrees. Combine the olive oil, chili powder, and pumpkin seeds in a medium bowl. Mix thoroughly, and place on an 11 by 17-inch baking sheet. Bake for 1 hour, stirring occasionally. Let cool on baking sheet before serving.

Recipe Notes

- Sprinkle in Pumpkin Black Bean Soup, Rosemary Split Pea Soup, or Zucchini Soup.
- Use as a salad topping.
- To make garlic-flavored seeds, subsititute the chili powder with ½ teaspoon garlic powder, ½ teaspoon onion powder, and ¼ teaspoon salt.

Pepitas are hulled pumpkin seeds. They are flat, dark-green seeds with a chewy texture and nutty flavor. Unhulled pumpkin seeds are covered by a white husk. Pepitas can be found in most health food stores and some supermarkets.

Spinach-Artichoke Dip

8 ounces firm tofu, drained

1 cup chopped canned artichokes, drained; reserve 2 tablespoons canned juices

½ (10-ounce) package frozen chopped spinach, thawed, squeezed dry

1 teaspoon dried basil

1 teaspoon salt

⅛ teaspoon pepper

2 teaspoons extra-virgin olive oil

¼ cup diced onion

2 cloves garlic, minced

YIELD: 8 servings
SERVING SIZE:
about ¼ cup

Preheat oven to 375 degrees. Place tofu, artichokes, artichoke juice, and spinach in a food processor or blender. Process until smooth. Transfer mixture to a medium bowl. Stir in basil, salt, and pepper. Set aside.

Heat oil in a small skillet, and cook onions and garlic until onions are translucent. Remove from heat, and stir into spinach-artichoke mixture. Place in a 3-cup glass or ceramic baking dish that has been rubbed with olive oil. Bake 20 minutes, or until edges start to brown. Serve warm.

Recipe Notes
- Serve with Tortilla Chips.
- Stir into cooked brown rice to make a casserole.
- Use as a spread for Whole Grain Tortillas.
- Works great as a sauce for Flatbread Pizza with Macadamia Nut Cheese.

Spinach and artichokes are made for each other. Not only do they taste great together, they're also extremely good for you. Spinach is an excellent source of vitamins and minerals, making it very nutrient dense. This heart-healthy food is loaded with bioflavonoids, which are plant organic compounds that act as antioxidants. Antioxidants protect the body from free radicals. Researchers have discovered at least thirteen different flavonoid compounds in spinach that aid in the prevention of disease.

Artichokes are high in fiber, potassium, calcium, iron, and phosphorus. They're also packed with antioxidants and phytonutrients, such as cynarin and silymarin. Cynarin stimulates digestion, protects the liver, and lowers triglycerides and cholesterol. Silymarin helps to prevent or reverse liver damage.

Taco Seasoning

YIELD: 48 servings
SERVING SIZE:
¼ teaspoon

2 tablespoons chili powder

1 tablespoon cumin

1 teaspoon garlic powder

1 teaspoon paprika

1 teaspoon onion powder
½ teaspoon oregano
⅛ teaspoon cayenne pepper

Mix all ingredients together and store in an airtight container.

Recipe Notes
- Adjust ingredient amounts according to preference.
- Add chipotle chili pepper seasoning for a smoky flavor.

> It's takes only a few minutes to make your own taco seasoning. Plus, you will save money, and it's much healthier for you. Store-bought taco seasoning usually contains sugar and preservatives and is loaded with sodium.

Tomato Slices with Avocado and Basil

2 medium tomatoes, unpeeled, unseeded, cut into 4 slices each
1 avocado, peeled, pitted, and sliced in 8 slices
Chopped fresh basil or dried basil, to taste
Salt, to taste

YIELD: 4 servings
SERVING SIZE:
   2 tomato slices and
   2 avocado slices

Place avocado slices on tomatoes and sprinkle with basil and salt.

Recipe Notes
- Use fresh oregano instead of basil.
- Drizzle Italian Salad Dressing over tomato slices.
- Add lettuce to make a salad.
- Sprinkle fresh lemon or lime juice over avocado slices to prevent browning if not serving immediately.

> To make avocado slices, cut avocado in half lengthwise and remove the seed. With a large spoon, scoop out the flesh in one piece and slice horizontally into strips.

Tortilla Chips

YIELD: 4 – 6 servings
SERVING SIZE:
8 – 12 chips

1 cup yellow cornmeal

½ cup warm water

½ tablespoon fresh lime juice

½ teaspoon salt

⅛ teaspoon pepper

Combine all ingredients in a bowl. Stir mixture until dough forms a ball and holds together. (It will be a wet dough.) Add a little water if necessary, a tablespoon or two at a time. Cover bowl with plastic wrap, and let dough rest at room temperature for 30 minutes.

Preheat oven to 400 degrees. Using your hands, press dough out onto an ungreased 11 by 17-inch baking sheet, making it as thin as possible. Use a knife to cut chips into 2-inch squares. Bake 20 minutes, or until slightly browned and crispy.

Recipe Notes

- Serve with Black Bean Dip, Confetti Hummus, Green Salsa Bean Dip, Hummus, Salsa, or Spinach-Artichoke Dip.
- Break chips into smaller pieces to garnish a bowl of soup.
- Add Taco Seasoning or chili powder to make spicy tortilla chips.

The triangular-shaped tortilla chip was popularized in the late 1940s by the owners of a Mexican tortilla factory in southwest Los Angeles. They found a way to make use of misshapen tortillas rejected from the automated tortilla manufacturing machine by cutting them into triangles and frying them.

Trail Mix

1 cup whole raw almonds or Cinnamon Roasted Almonds (p. 85)
1 cup cashew halves and pieces
1 cup walnut halves and pieces
½ cup golden raisins
½ cup raisins
¼ cup raw sunflower seeds
¼ cup raw pumpkin seeds (pepitas)

YIELD: 12 servings
SERVING SIZE:
about ¼ cup

Mix all ingredients together and store in an airtight container for 2 weeks at room temperature or 1 month in refrigerator.

Recipe Notes
• Use as a topping for fresh fruit.
• Serve with almond milk for a quick breakfast dish.
• Other dried fruit options are apricots, bananas, blueberries, dates, or figs.
• Other nut options are Brazil nuts, macadamia nuts, or pecans.
• Add unsweetened coconut flakes.

Trail Mix is the ideal snack when you're traveling or on the go. Plan ahead by measuring out your appropriate serving size, and place in a plastic zip-top bag. Take your Trail Mix to work, to school, in the car, or on an airplane. That way, when you're away from home, you won't be tempted by foods that don't fit within the Daniel Fast guidelines.

Appetizers and Snacks

Salads and Salad Dressings

Salads

Salad Dressings

Blackberry, Avocado, and Mango Salad

4 cups mixed salad greens, loosely packed
1 cup blackberries
1 ripe avocado, peeled, pitted, and cut into 1-inch cubes
1 cup mango, pitted, and cut into 1-inch cubes
½ cup pecan halves
1 recipe Orange–Poppy Seed Salad Dressing (p. 116)

YIELD: 4 servings
SERVING SIZE:
about 1½ cups

In a large bowl, combine salad greens, blackberries, avocado, mango, and pecan halves. Toss, and serve with Orange–Poppy Seed Salad Dressing.

Recipe Notes
• Substitute mango with 1 cup peaches, peeled, pitted, and chopped into 1-inch cubes.

Butternut Squash and Broccoli Salad

1½ pounds butternut squash, peeled and cut into 1-inch cubes (about 3 cups)
3 cups chopped broccoli florets, cut into 1-inch pieces
½ cup canned black beans, rinsed and drained
1½ tablespoons extra-virgin olive oil
2 tablespoons chopped fresh parsley
¼ teaspoon dried basil
¼ teaspoon garlic powder
⅛ teaspoon thyme
2 tablespoons toasted chopped walnuts for garnish
2 tablespoons toasted pumpkin seeds (pepitas) for garnish

YIELD: 4 servings
SERVING SIZE:
about 1¼ cups

Using a vegetable steamer, cook butternut squash about 5 minutes. Add broccoli, and cook another 12 minutes. Vegetables should be crisp tender. Remove from steamer, and place in a large bowl. Add black beans. In a separate smaller bowl, whisk together oil, parsley, basil, garlic powder, and thyme. Pour over vegetables and beans, and mix well. Serve warm, or let sit at room temperature for 10–15 minutes. Just before serving, sprinkle walnuts and pumpkin seeds on top.

Recipe Notes
- This dish is best served warm, but it can also be eaten cold, straight out of the refrigerator.
- Use as a topping for a lettuce salad.

> The dressing for this salad is very mild, just enough to give it a hint of flavor. Use garlic powder instead of fresh garlic to avoid overpowering the flavor of the vegetables.

Fig, Pear, and Walnut Salad

YIELD: 4 servings
SERVING SIZE:
about 1 cup

4 cups torn romaine lettuce, loosely packed
1 Bosc pear, unpeeled, sliced thin
¼ cup diced dried figs
¼ cup chopped walnuts
2 tablespoons raw sunflower seeds
1 recipe Apple-Cinnamon Salad Dressing (p. 113)

Place 1 cup of greens on each plate. Arrange pear slices on top of each mound of lettuce. Sprinkle each salad with 1 tablespoon figs, 1 tablespoon walnuts, and ½ tablespoon sunflower seeds. Drizzle about 2 tablespoons dressing over each salad.

Recipe Notes
- Use an apple instead of a pear, or try a combination of both.
- Serve with mixed greens or fresh spinach.
- Substitute pecans for the walnuts.

> Figs are teardrop-shaped fruits that are sweet, succulent, and chewy. However, since their skins are delicate and prone to perish quickly, figs often are dried. Two of the most popular types of figs are Black Mission and Calimyrna.

Marinated Vegetable Salad

  1 recipe Marinated Zucchini (p. 150)
  2 cups broccoli florets, cut into bite-size pieces
1½ cups diced carrots
  2 tablespoons chopped fresh parsley (optional)

YIELD: 8 servings
SERVING SIZE:
  about ½ cup

Prepare Marinated Zucchini as directed and place in a large bowl. Steam or boil broccoli and carrots until crisp tender. Add broccoli and carrots (drain first, if boiled) to zucchini and stir well. Add parsley, if desired. Cover and let sit at room temperature for 1 hour.

Recipe Notes
- Add artichokes, cooked sweet peas, mushrooms, black olives, and/or roasted red bell peppers.
- This dish is best when made ahead of time and refrigerated overnight. Bring to room temperature before serving.

Vegetables that are lightly steamed (5–15 minutes, depending on the vegetable) rather than overcooked on the stovetop or grill retain most of their vitamins and are easier to digest. Steaming also brings out the natural sugars in the vegetables, which intensifies their flavors.

Mediterranean Black Bean Salad

  2 (15-ounce) cans black beans, rinsed and drained
  1 cup chopped green bell peppers
  1 cup chopped red bell peppers
  1 cup chopped tomatoes, unpeeled, unseeded
  1 cup chopped avocado, cut into ½-inch cubes (about 1 medium avocado)
  ½ cup diced onion
  ¼ cup chopped fresh parsley or cilantro

YIELD: 12 servings
SERVING SIZE:
  about ½ cup

Dressing
  2 tablespoons fresh lime juice
  1 tablespoon extra-virgin olive oil
  2 cloves garlic, minced
  ½ teaspoon salt

Put beans, peppers, tomatoes, avocado, onions, and parsley in a large bowl. In a small bowl, combine lime juice, olive oil, garlic, and salt. Whisk until combined and pour over salad. Toss well to coat. Refrigerate 2 – 4 hours to allow flavors to blend, and serve.

Recipe Notes
- If you don't have fresh parsley on hand, use 1 teaspoon of dried parsley.
- Serve over romaine or spinach leaves.

> Brightly colored bell peppers, whether green, red, orange, or yellow, are excellent sources of vitamin A and vitamin C, two very powerful antioxidants.

Mega Greek Salad

YIELD: 6 servings
SERVING SIZE: about 1 cup

4 cups torn romaine lettuce
1 cup chopped canned artichokes, drained
1 cup sliced cherry tomatoes
1 cup quartered cucumber slices, peeled
1 cup sliced black olives
½ cup diced green bell pepper
½ cup sliced red onion
½ cup chopped fresh parsley

Dressing
¼ cup extra-virgin olive oil
¼ cup fresh lemon juice
2 teaspoons dried oregano flakes
½ teaspoon salt
⅛ teaspoon pepper

Put lettuce in a large bowl. Add artichokes, cherry tomatoes, cucumbers, olives, peppers, onions, and parsley.

In a small bowl, combine olive oil, lemon juice, oregano, salt, and pepper. Just before serving, whisk until well combined and pour over salad. Toss to coat and serve.

Recipe Notes

- If you don't have fresh parsley on hand for the salad, add 1 teaspoon dried parsley to the salad dressing.

A traditional Greek salad typically contains chunks of feta cheese. However, you won't even miss the feta in this fantastic salad!

Ozarks Sunset Fruit Salad

2 cups torn fresh spinach leaves, packed, stems removed
2 cups torn romaine lettuce, packed
2 cups orange segments, cut into 1-inch pieces
2 kiwifruit, peeled and cut into half moons
1 cup sliced strawberries
½ cup blueberries
¼ cup sliced or slivered almonds, toasted

YIELD: 4 servings
SERVING SIZE:
about 1¼ cups

Place ingredients in a large bowl and toss to combine. Serve with choice of dressing.

Recipe Notes

- Serve with Orange–Poppy Seed Salad Dressing or Apple-Cinnamon Salad Dressing.

The inspiration for this colorful fruit salad came a few summers ago when I was sitting on my back deck watching the sun dip below the horizon. The sky was an amazing display of color, so beautiful and vibrant. As I saw that majestic scene unfold, I was overwhelmed with the thought that the God who created that incredible Ozarks sunset is also deeply in love with me.

Salads and Salad Dressings

Quinoa Salad

1½ cups cooked quinoa

½ cup diced cucumber

½ cup chopped sugar snap peas

½ cup diced tomato

½ cup diced orange bell pepper

½ cup diced yellow bell pepper

¼ cup grated carrot

¼ cup pine nuts

2 tablespoons chopped fresh basil

2 tablespoons chopped fresh parsley

1 recipe Italian Salad Dressing (p. 115)

Mixed greens (optional)

Mix quinoa, vegetables, pine nuts, basil, and parsley. Pour Italian Salad Dressing over all. Stir well to combine. Serve alone or with mixed greens.

Recipe Notes

• Experiment with different combinations of vegetables. Try artichokes, broccoli, celery, black olives, or steamed asparagus.

• Add chickpeas.

• Use chopped walnuts instead of pine nuts.

• Sprinkle sunflower and/or pumpkin seeds (pepitas) on top.

• Substitute Lemon-Tahini Salad Dressing for Italian Salad Dressing.

Quinoa (pronounced "KEEN-wa") is a tiny seed that packs a powerful protein punch for its size. It's a complete protein, since it contains all nine essential amino acids. Though quinoa appears to be a grain and is often mistaken for one, it's actually the seed from a leafy plant. Quinoa is also high in fiber and is easily digested.

To cook quinoa, pour 1 cup into a fine mesh strainer over the sink, and rinse with cold water. Place in a medium saucepan, and add 1½ cups water. Bring to a boil. Reduce heat to low and cover. Simmer gently with lid tilted for 15 minutes or until nearly all of the liquid is absorbed. Remove from heat and let sit for 5 minutes with the lid on. Makes about 3 cups cooked quinoa.

Roasted Potato Salad

YIELD: 4 servings
SERVING SIZE:
about 1 cup

- 1 pound B-size red potatoes, unpeeled
- ½ pound Brussels sprouts, trimmed and halved
- 1 cup trimmed fresh green beans, cut into 1-inch pieces
- 1½ tablespoons extra-virgin olive oil, divided
- ½ teaspoon tarragon
- ½ teaspoon salt
- ⅛ teaspoon pepper
- ¼ cup chopped red onion
- ¼ cup finely chopped pecans or walnuts
- 2 cups chopped romaine lettuce

Scrub potatoes well. Place in a large saucepan, and cover with water. Heat to boiling. Reduce heat slightly to a soft rolling boil, and cook, uncovered, 15 minutes. Drain, and allow to cool for 10 minutes.

Preheat oven to 425 degrees. Cut potatoes into quarters, and place in a large bowl, along with Brussels sprouts and green beans. Add 1 tablespoon olive oil, tarragon, salt, and pepper. Stir well to coat. Place vegetables on an 11 by 17-inch baking sheet. Bake 10 minutes, and flip. Cook another 10 minutes, or until vegetables are slightly browned. Place in a large bowl, and set aside.

Heat ½ tablespoon olive oil in skillet over medium heat. Add onions and pecans, and cook until onions are soft and translucent. Mix with potatoes and vegetables. To serve, place ½ cup lettuce on each plate, and top with roasted potato-vegetable mixture.

Recipe Notes
- You can also use frozen Brussels sprouts and frozen green beans for this recipe. Lightly steam or slightly undercook them in boiling water before roasting.
- Substitute chopped asparagus spears for the green beans.
- Use fresh spinach instead of romaine lettuce.

A member of the cabbage family, Brussels sprouts are high in vitamin A, vitamin C, calcium, and potassium. They're also a good source of fiber, containing 3–5 grams of fiber per cup. Unlike most vegetables, Brussels sprouts are high in protein.

Spinach Salad

YIELD: 4 servings
SERVING SIZE:
about 1 cup

4 cups torn fresh spinach, loosely packed
1 cup canned chickpeas, rinsed and drained
1 cup chopped carrots
1 cup chopped sugar snap peas
1 cup chopped tomatoes, unpeeled, unseeded
1 cup chopped zucchini
2 tablespoons raw sunflower seeds

Place spinach, chickpeas, carrots, sugar snap peas, tomatoes, and zucchini in a large bowl. Sprinkle in sunflower seeds, and toss gently. Serve with choice of dressing.

Recipe Notes
• Serve with Avocado-Tomato Salad Dressing, Italian Salad Dressing, or Lemon-Tahini Salad Dressing.

Sunflower seeds are an excellent source of vitamin E, the body's primary fat-soluble antioxidant.

Strawberry-Spinach Salad

YIELD: 4 servings
SERVING SIZE:
about 1½ cups

4 cups torn fresh spinach leaves, packed, stems removed
2 cups sliced strawberries
4 teaspoons raw sunflower seeds
1 teaspoon sesame seeds
½ teaspoon poppy seeds
1 recipe Apple-Cinnamon Salad Dressing (p. 113)

Place 1 cup spinach and ½ cup strawberries on each salad plate. Sprinkle each serving with 1 teaspoon sunflower seeds, ¼ teaspoon sesame seeds, and ⅛ teaspoon poppy seeds. Drizzle Apple-Cinnamon Salad Dressing over all and serve.

Strawberries are very perishable, so they shouldn't be washed until right before eating or using in a recipe. Do not remove their caps and stems until after you have washed them under cold running water and patted them dry. This will prevent the berries from absorbing excess water, which can negatively affect their flavor.

Taco Salad

1 (14.5-ounce) can corn kernels, drained
1 (15-ounce) can pinto beans, undrained
¼ teaspoon garlic powder
¼ teaspoon salt
1 tablespoon extra-virgin olive oil
½ cup diced onion
1 (15-ounce) can black beans, rinsed and drained
½ tablespoon Taco Seasoning (p. 98)
2 cups chopped romaine lettuce or iceberg lettuce

YIELD: 4 servings
SERVING SIZE:
about 1½ cups

Toppings

Avocado slices, diced green onions, sliced black olives, diced tomatoes

Preheat oven to 425 degrees. Spread corn kernels out in one layer on a lightly oiled 11 by 17-inch baking sheet. Bake for 20–25 minutes, or until browned and slightly crunchy.

While corn is roasting, place pinto beans in a small saucepan over medium heat. Add garlic powder and salt. Cook 10 minutes, stirring occasionally. Using a fork or potato masher, mash beans until they are the consistency of refried beans. Lower heat, and continue to cook until some of the liquid has evaporated and beans have thickened, about 10 minutes more. Stir frequently to avoid scalding beans on the bottom of the pan.

Heat olive oil in a large skillet over medium heat and add onions. Cook until onions are soft and translucent. Add black beans, corn, and Taco Seasoning. Stir well to coat beans with olive oil and seasonings. Reduce heat to low and keep warm until pinto beans are done.

Salads and Salad Dressings

To serve, place about ½ cup lettuce on a plate, and top with ¼ cup pinto beans and a heaping ½ cup of black-bean-and-corn mixture. Add desired toppings to salad.

Recipe Notes

- Serve with Tortilla Chips.
- Instead of roasting the corn kernels, use them straight out of the can.
- Use as filling in Whole Grain Tortillas.
- Top each serving with 2 tablespoons Salsa.

> Oven-roasting the corn gives it a crunchier texture and a slightly sweeter taste.

Tomato, Fennel, and Cucumber Salad

YIELD: 8 servings
SERVING SIZE:
about ½ cup

1 pint cherry or grape tomatoes, halved (about 3 cups)
1 cup diced cucumbers, peeled
1 cup chopped fennel bulb
¼ cup chopped green onion
2 tablespoons chopped fresh parsley
1 tablespoon extra-virgin olive oil
¼ teaspoon toasted fennel seeds

Combine all ingredients in a large bowl. Refrigerate 2 – 4 hours. Serve chilled.

Recipe Notes

- Add chopped fresh basil.
- Mix in cubed avocado.
- Substitute raw sunflower seeds for fennel seeds.
- Serve on top of chopped romaine lettuce or spinach.
- Drizzle with Italian Salad Dressing.

> Fennel seeds taste like licorice and are often used in Italian cooking. They have been known to soothe digestive problems, and in some countries, they are served as an after-meal breath freshener.

White Bean Salad

4 cups torn romaine lettuce, packed
1 cup canned cannellini beans, rinsed and drained
1 cup chopped sugar snap peas
1 cup halved cherry or grape tomatoes
2 tablespoons chopped red onion
2 tablespoons chopped fresh basil
2 tablespoons chopped fresh parsley

YIELD: 4 servings
SERVING SIZE:
  about 1½ cups

Place lettuce in a large bowl and add beans, sugar snap peas, tomatoes, onions, basil, and parsley. Toss, and serve with choice of dressing.

Recipe Notes
• Serve with Avocado-Tomato Salad Dressing, Italian Salad Dressing, or Lemon-Tahini Salad Dressing.
• Use spinach or mixed greens instead of romaine lettuce.
• Substitute cooked, cooled chopped asparagus, green beans, or sweet peas for the sugar snap peas.
• Add ¼ cup raw sunflower seeds.

> Cannellini beans, or white kidney beans, are similar in color and shape to great northern beans, and can be substituted for great northern beans in most recipes that call for them.

Apple-Cinnamon Salad Dressing

¼ cup extra-virgin olive oil
¼ cup unsweetened apple juice
1 tablespoon fresh lemon juice
1 tablespoon diced red onion
¼ teaspoon cinnamon

YIELD: 8 servings
SERVING SIZE:
  about 1 tablespoon

Combine all ingredients in a covered glass jar, and shake well. Refrigerate until ready to use.

Recipe Notes
- Use as a dressing for Ozarks Sunset Fruit Salad or Strawberry-Spinach Salad.
- Drizzle over fresh fruit.

> Cinnamon is available in either stick or powder form. It should be kept in a cool, dark, and dry place. Ground cinnamon will keep for about six months, while cinnamon sticks will stay fresh for about one year stored this way. You can extend their shelf life by keeping them in the refrigerator. To check whether cinnamon is still fresh, smell it. If it does not smell sweet, it should be discarded.

Avocado-Tomato Salad Dressing

YIELD: 16 servings
SERVING SIZE:
about 1 tablespoon

1 avocado, pitted
1 cup chopped tomatoes, unpeeled, unseeded
2 tablespoons extra-virgin olive oil
1 clove garlic, minced
2 tablespoons chopped fresh parsley or 1½ teaspoons dried parsley
1 tablespoon chopped fresh basil or 1 teaspoon dried basil
¼ teaspoon salt

Cut avocado in half and remove the seed. Use a large spoon to scoop out the flesh. Mix in a blender with all remaining ingredients. Blend until smooth. Makes 1 cup.

Recipe Notes
- Use as a dressing for Spinach Salad or any lettuce salad.
- Serve with fresh vegetables.
- Add water if you desire a thinner dressing.

> A firm avocado will ripen in a paper bag at room temperature within a few days. As the fruit ripens, the skin will turn darker. Avocados should not be refrigerated until they are ripe. Once ripe, they can be kept refrigerated for up to a week.

Italian Salad Dressing

½ cup extra-virgin olive oil

2 tablespoons fresh lemon juice

1 clove garlic, minced

1 teaspoon dried basil

½ teaspoon dried oregano flakes

¼ teaspoon salt

YIELD: 8 servings
SERVING SIZE:
  about 1 tablespoon

Place all ingredients in a blender and mix to combine. Refrigerate until chilled.

Recipe Notes

• Serve with Quinoa Salad, Spinach Salad, or White Bean Salad.

• Use with any lettuce salad.

• Drizzle over Tomato Slices with Avocado and Basil.

> When it comes to cooking, not all oils are created equal. Olive oil is one of the most heart-healthy choices because the monounsaturated fat it contains can help to reduce the risk of heart disease by lowering cholesterol levels in the blood. When selecting an olive oil, be sure to choose extra-virgin, because it is the least processed.

Lemon-Tahini Salad Dressing

¼ cup extra-virgin olive oil

2 tablespoons fresh lemon juice

2 tablespoons tahini

1 clove garlic, minced

1 tablespoon chopped fresh basil or ½ teaspoon dried basil

1 tablespoon chopped fresh parsley or ½ teaspoon dried parsley

YIELD: 8 servings
SERVING SIZE:
  about 1 tablespoon

Place all ingredients in a blender and mix. Refrigerate until chilled.

Salads and Salad Dressings

Recipe Notes
- Use as a dressing for Quinoa Salad, Spinach Salad, White Bean Salad, or any lettuce salad.
- Tahini is a thick paste made from ground sesame seeds. It is a staple in Middle Eastern cooking and can be found at health food stores and most large grocery chains.

> Lemons will stay fresh when kept at room temperature away from exposure to sunlight for about a week. If you won't be using them within this time period, you can store lemons in the refrigerator crisper, where they will keep for about four weeks.

Orange - Poppy Seed Salad Dressing

YIELD: 8 servings
SERVING SIZE:
  about 1 tablespoon

¼ cup extra-virgin olive oil
¼ cup orange juice
2 tablespoons fresh lemon juice
1 tablespoon diced red onion
½ teaspoon poppy seeds
¼ teaspoon grated orange zest
⅛ teaspoon dry mustard
⅛ teaspoon salt

Combine all ingredients in a covered glass jar, and shake well. Refrigerate until ready to use.

Recipe Notes
- Serve with Blackberry, Avocado, and Mango Salad or Ozarks Sunset Fruit Salad
- Use with any lettuce salad.

> The zest is the outermost, colorful skin of citrus fruits. Zest is often used to enhance flavor in recipes. The pith, or white membrane underneath the outside peel, has a bitter, unpleasant taste and should be avoided while zesting.

Soups

Black-and-White Chili

YIELD: 8 servings
SERVING SIZE:
  about 1 cup

1 tablespoon extra-virgin olive oil

1 cup chopped onion

1 clove garlic, minced

4 cups water or Vegetable Broth (p. 134)

3 (15-ounce) cans black beans, rinsed and drained

3 (15-ounce) can great northern beans, rinsed and drained

1 tablespoon chili powder

½ teaspoon cumin

½ teaspoon salt

Heat olive oil in a large saucepan over medium heat. Stir in onions, and cook until soft and translucent. Add garlic, and cook for 30 seconds, stirring constantly so garlic doesn't burn. Add water or broth, beans, chili powder, cumin, and salt. Heat to boiling. Reduce heat, and simmer uncovered for 30 minutes.

Recipe Notes
• Use navy beans instead of great northern beans.
• Serve with Corn Muffins or Tortilla Chips.

Rinsing and draining canned beans helps to remove the added sodium.

Black Bean Minestrone

YIELD: **6 servings**
SERVING SIZE:
  about 1¼ cups

- 1 tablespoon extra-virgin olive oil
- ½ cup chopped onion
- 1 cup chopped carrots
- 2 stalks celery, sliced
- 2 cloves garlic, minced
- 4 cups water or Vegetable Broth (p. 134)
- 1 (15-ounce) can black beans, rinsed and drained
- 1 cup fresh or frozen green beans, cut into 1-inch pieces
- 1 cup chopped tomatoes, unpeeled, unseeded
- 1 cup chopped fresh spinach or ½ cup frozen spinach, thawed
- 2 tablespoons chopped fresh basil or 1½ teaspoons dried basil
- 2 tablespoons chopped fresh parsley or 1½ teaspoons dried parsley
- ½ teaspoon salt
- ⅛ teaspoon pepper

Heat olive oil in a large saucepan over medium heat. Cook onions, carrots, and celery until vegetables are softened. Stir in garlic, and cook for 30 seconds, stirring constantly so garlic doesn't burn.

Add water or broth, black beans, green beans, tomatoes, spinach, basil, salt, and pepper. Bring to a boil. Simmer, uncovered, over low heat about 20 minutes to allow the flavors to blend. Stir in parsley just before serving.

Recipe Notes
- Serve with Broiled Polenta Squares or Corn Muffins.
- Add barley, brown rice, or whole grain pasta.
- Other vegetables to add: corn, peas, potatoes, squash, and/or zucchini.
- For more tomato flavor, add ½ cup tomato sauce.
- Use 1 (14.5-ounce) can undrained diced tomatoes instead of fresh tomatoes.

Minestrone comes from the Italian word *minestra*, which refers to chunky soup. Minestrone soups are generally tomato based with beans, onions, celery, crushed or chopped tomatoes, and carrots.

Black-Eyed Peas and Potato Soup

YIELD: 6 servings
SERVING SIZE:
about 1 cup

1 tablespoon extra-virgin olive oil
1 cup chopped onion
1 cup sliced carrots
1 cup chopped celery
2 cloves garlic, minced
4 cups water or Vegetable Broth (p. 134)
1 (15-ounce) can black-eyed peas, rinsed and drained
2 cups cubed russet potatoes, peeled
2 tablespoons chopped fresh parsley or 2 teaspoons dried parsley
½ tablespoon dried chives
½ teaspoon salt
⅛ teaspoon cayenne pepper
⅛ teaspoon pepper

Heat olive oil in a large saucepan over medium heat. Add onions, carrots, and celery. Cook until vegetables are softened. Stir in garlic, and cook for 30 seconds, stirring constantly so garlic doesn't burn. Add water or broth, black-eyed peas, potatoes, parsley, chives, salt, cayenne pepper, and pepper. Bring to a boil. Reduce heat, cover, and simmer 30 minutes.

Recipe Notes
• Instead of black-eyed peas, use great northern beans, cannellini beans, or navy beans.

Black-eyed peas are small ivory-colored beans that have a black dot on one side.

Butternut Squash and Sweet Potato Soup

½ tablespoon extra-virgin olive oil

½ cup chopped onion

4 cups water or Vegetable Broth (p. 134)

1 pound butternut squash, peeled and cut into 1-inch cubes

1 pound sweet potatoes, peeled and cut into 1-inch cubes

1 teaspoon fresh minced ginger root or ½ teaspoon ground ginger

½ teaspoon salt

⅛ teaspoon allspice

⅛ teaspoon cinnamon

⅛ teaspoon nutmeg

YIELD: **6 servings**
SERVING SIZE:
about 1 cup

Heat olive oil in large saucepan over medium heat, and add onions. Cook until onions are soft and translucent. Add water or broth and remaining ingredients to saucepan, and bring to a boil. Reduce heat, and cover. Simmer 30 minutes or until vegetables are tender.

Remove vegetables with a slotted spoon and place in a food processor or blender. Puree until smooth. (You may need to do this in two batches, because filling your processor or blender more than half full could cause the hot soup to pop the lid.) Return to heat, and stir well. Use a whisk, if necessary, to smooth out the texture. Cook another 5 – 10 minutes, and serve.

Recipe Notes

• If you prefer a chunkier texture, pulse the vegetables a few times instead of pureeing them.

• Use chopped leeks instead of onions (light green and white parts only).

Butternut squash is an hourglass-shaped winter squash. It has a tough, inedible skin and a deep orange-colored flesh that tastes sweet.

Carrot, Apple, and Ginger Soup

YIELD: 8 servings
SERVING SIZE:
about 1 cup

½ tablespoon extra-virgin olive oil
½ cup chopped onion
1 clove garlic, minced
1 tablespoon minced fresh ginger root
6 cups water or Vegetable Broth (p. 134)
2 pounds carrots, peeled and cut into 2-inch pieces
2 cups chopped apples, peeled
1 bay leaf
½ teaspoon dried thyme
1 teaspoon salt

Heat olive oil over medium heat in a large saucepan or stockpot. Add onions, and cook until soft and translucent. Mix in garlic and ginger root. Cook for 30 seconds, stirring constantly. Add water or broth, carrots, apples, bay leaf, thyme, and salt. Bring to a boil. Reduce heat, and cover. Simmer 20 minutes, or until carrots are tender. When done, discard bay leaf.

Puree the soup in batches in a food processor or blender, being careful not to fill more than half full at a time (so the hot soup doesn't pop the lid). When smooth, return to stovetop and cook another 10 minutes.

Recipe Notes
• If you like this combination of flavors and have a juicer, try the Orient Express.
• Use 1 teaspoon dried ginger if you don't have fresh ginger root.

To remove the skin from fresh mature ginger, peel it with a paring knife. The ginger can then be sliced, minced, or julienned.

Chipotle Chili

1 tablespoon extra-virgin olive oil

1 cup chopped red onion

2 cloves garlic, minced

2 cups water or Vegetable Broth (p. 134)

1 (15-ounce) can black beans, rinsed and drained

1 (15-ounce) can cannellini beans, rinsed and drained

1 (15-ounce) can dark red kidney beans, rinsed and drained

1 (15-ounce) can pinto beans, rinsed and drained

1 (14.5-ounce) can diced tomatoes, undrained

1 tablespoon fresh lime juice

1 teaspoon chipotle chili pepper seasoning

1 teaspoon salt

YIELD: 8 servings
SERVING SIZE:
   about 1 cup

Heat olive oil in a large, deep skillet or saucepan. Add onions, and cook until soft and translucent. Stir in garlic, and cook for 30 seconds, stirring constantly so garlic doesn't burn. Add water or broth, beans, tomatoes, lime juice, chipotle chili pepper, and salt. Bring to a boil. Reduce heat, and simmer, covered, for 30 minutes.

Recipe Notes
• Serve with Broiled Polenta Squares or Tortilla Chips.
• Add 1 cup cooked brown rice.

A lime will produce more juice when kept at room temperature. If refrigerated, place lime in a bowl of warm water for several minutes. Before slicing, roll lime under the palm of your hand on a flat surface to extract juice.

Chunky Potato Soup

YIELD: 6 servings
SERVING SIZE:
about 1 cup

1 tablespoon extra-virgin olive oil
½ cup chopped onion
1 cup chopped carrots
1 cup chopped celery
2 cloves garlic, minced
4 cups water or Vegetable Broth (p. 134)
3 large russet potatoes, peeled, cubed (about 5 cups)
1 bay leaf
1 teaspoon salt
½ teaspoon thyme
⅛ teaspoon pepper
½ cup unsweetened almond milk
2 tablespoons chopped fresh parsley or 1 teaspoon dried parsley

Heat olive oil in saucepan over medium heat. Cook onions, carrots, and celery until vegetables are softened. Stir in garlic, and cook for 30 seconds, stirring constantly so garlic doesn't burn.

Add water or broth, potatoes, bay leaf, salt, thyme, and pepper. Bring to a boil. Simmer, covered, for 30 minutes or until potatoes are tender. Discard bay leaf. Add half of potato mixture to a food processor or blender, and process until smooth. (You may need to do this in two batches, because filling your processor or blender more than half full could cause the hot soup to pop the lid.) Return to saucepan. Stir in almond milk and parsley. Cook until heated through, and serve.

Recipe Notes
• Sprinkle diced green onions on top of each serving.
• Make this a creamy soup by putting the whole potato mixture into a food processor or blender.
• Use rice milk or soy milk instead of almond milk.

> White potatoes are a carbohydrate-rich food, and although that is often viewed as a bad thing, potatoes are actually quite good for you. Their complex carbohydrates supply the body with its main source of fuel for energy. Potatoes are also high in fiber, potassium, and vitamin C.

Cinnamon-Cumin Lentil Soup

6 cups water or Vegetable Broth (p. 134)

1 cup dry lentils, sorted and rinsed

1 (15-ounce) can chickpeas, rinsed and drained

½ cup diced carrots

½ cup diced red onion

½ teaspoon cinnamon

½ teaspoon cumin

¼ teaspoon salt

YIELD: 6 servings
SERVING SIZE:
about 1 cup

Bring water or broth to a boil. Add lentils, chickpeas, carrots, onions, cinnamon, cumin, and salt. Simmer gently with lid tilted for 30 minutes, and serve.

Recipe Notes

- To sort lentils, spread them in a single layer on an 11 by 17-inch baking sheet. Look for discolored and misshapen beans, and discard any unwanted debris. Place good lentils into a colander and rinse thoroughly using cold water.
- Add cooked brown or wild rice to the soup.
- Puree half of the soup by putting it in a food processor.

It might not seem likely that cinnamon and cumin would go well together, but they really do complement each other nicely in this hearty lentil soup.

Jamaican Chili

YIELD: 4 servings
SERVING SIZE:
about 1¼ cups

1   tablespoon extra-virgin olive oil
1   cup chopped onion
1½ cups chopped yellow bell pepper, seeded
2   cloves garlic, minced
1   cup water or Vegetable Broth (p. 134)
1   (15-ounce) can black beans, rinsed and drained
1   (15-ounce) can cannellini beans, rinsed and drained
1   (15-ounce) can kidney beans, rinsed and drained
1   (14.5-ounce) can diced tomatoes, undrained
1   teaspoon cumin
1   teaspoon paprika
½   teaspoon salt
¼   cup chopped fresh parsley

Heat olive oil in large saucepan over medium heat, and cook onions until soft and translucent. Add yellow pepper and garlic. Cook until pepper is tender, stirring frequently. Add water or broth, beans, tomatoes, cumin, paprika, and salt. Bring to a boil. Cover, and simmer 30 minutes. Stir in parsley just before serving.

Recipe Notes
• For a spicier chili, add a diced jalapeno pepper or hot chili powder.
• Serve with Broiled Polenta Squares or Corn Muffins.
• Use chickpeas instead of cannellini beans.
• Add more vegetables, such as carrots, celery, or zucchini.

Paprika is a red spice made from dried bell peppers. Depending on how it was produced, the intensity of paprika's flavor can range from delicate to very hot. The deep red varieties tend to be sweeter, while the light brown-orange paprika is usually very spicy.

Pumpkin Black Bean Soup

1 tablespoon extra-virgin olive oil

1 cup chopped onion

2 cloves garlic, minced

4 cups water or Vegetable Broth (p. 134)

3 (15-ounce) cans black beans, rinsed and drained

1 (14.5-ounce) can diced tomatoes, undrained

1 (15-ounce) can pumpkin

1½ teaspoons cumin

1½ teaspoons salt

⅛ teaspoon pepper

Spicy Pumpkin Seeds (p. 97) (optional)

YIELD: 8 servings
SERVING SIZE:
about 1 cup

Heat olive oil in large saucepan over medium heat, and add onions. Cook until soft and translucent. Stir in garlic, and cook for 30 seconds, stirring constantly so garlic doesn't burn. Add water or broth, 2 cups of the black beans, pumpkin, cumin, salt, and pepper. Put tomatoes and remaining black beans into a food processor or blender until smooth. Add to soup mixture, and heat to boiling. Reduce heat, and simmer 30 minutes. Sprinkle Spicy Pumpkin Seeds on top of each serving.

Recipe Notes

• For a chunkier soup, put only 2 cups black beans into the food processor and keep the tomatoes diced.

• Use chili powder or Taco Seasoning in place of cumin.

> To make your own fresh pumpkin puree, cut a sugar pumpkin in half, remove the stem, and extract the seeds and strings. Place halves facedown in a baking dish. Add ½ inch warm water to pan to help keep the flesh moist.
>
> Bake at 450 degrees for 45 minutes to 1 hour, or until you can pierce the skin with a fork. Remove from oven and let sit until cool enough to handle. Scoop pumpkin flesh out with a spoon. Put flesh in a food processor until smooth, or mash with a potato masher. You may use this puree in any recipe that calls for canned pumpkin.

Rice, Bean, and Sweet Potato Soup

YIELD: 8 servings
SERVING SIZE:
  about 1¼ cups

8 cups water or Vegetable Broth (p. 134)

1 pound sweet potatoes (about 3 cups), peeled, diced

1 (15-ounce) can black beans, rinsed and drained

2 cups cooked brown rice

½ cup chopped celery

½ cup chopped onion

2 tablespoons chopped fresh parsley or 2 teaspoons dried parsley

1 bay leaf

1 teaspoon thyme

1 teaspoon salt

⅛ teaspoon pepper

Place all ingredients in a large stockpot. Heat to boiling. Reduce heat, and simmer 20 minutes. Discard bay leaf. Put half of soup in a food processor or blender and puree until smooth. (You may need to do this in two batches, because filling your processor or blender more than half full could cause the hot soup to pop the lid.) Return to stockpot, and cook 10 more minutes.

Recipe Notes
• Use cannellini beans, navy beans, or great northern beans instead of black beans.
• Substitute wild rice for brown rice or use a combination of both.

> The difference between brown rice and white rice is much more than just color. The process that produces brown rice removes only the outermost layer—the hull—of the rice kernel and is the least damaging to its nutritional value. The complete milling and polishing that converts brown rice into white rice destroys 67 percent of the vitamin B3, 80 percent of the vitamin B1, 90 percent of the vitamin B6, half of the manganese, half of the phosphorus, 60 percent of the iron, and all of the dietary fiber and essential fatty acids. The healthier choice is always brown rice over white rice.

Rosemary Split Pea Soup

1 tablespoon extra-virgin olive oil

1 cup sliced carrots

1 cup diced onion

2 cloves garlic, minced

6 cups water or Vegetable Broth (p. 134)

2 cups dry split peas

1 teaspoon dried crushed rosemary

1 bay leaf

1 teaspoon salt

YIELD: 6 servings
SERVING SIZE:
  about 1 cup

Empty split peas in a colander, and rinse well. Sort through peas to remove any unwanted particles. Set aside. Heat olive oil in large saucepan or stockpot over medium heat. Add carrots and onions. Cook until onions are soft and translucent. Stir in garlic, and cook 30 seconds, stirring constantly so garlic doesn't burn. Add water or broth, peas, rosemary, bay leaf, and salt. Heat to boiling, and then reduce heat to low. Simmer 30 minutes with lid on and slightly tilted.

Remove peas and vegetables, and discard bay leaf. Transfer to a food processor or blender. Process until smooth. (You may need to do this in two batches, because filling your processor or blender more than half full could cause the hot soup to pop the lid.) Return to saucepan. Cook 5 more minutes, and serve.

Recipe Notes
- Top with toasted pumpkin seeds (pepitas) and/or raw sunflower seeds.

Split peas are a good source of cholesterol-lowering fiber, which helps to stablize blood sugar levels.

Taco Soup

YIELD: 8 servings
SERVING SIZE:
about 1 cup

1 tablespoon extra-virgin olive oil

½ cup diced onion

4 cups water or Vegetable Broth (p. 134)

1 (14.5 ounce) can diced tomatoes, undrained

1 (15-ounce) can black beans, rinsed and drained

1 (15-ounce) can pinto beans, rinsed, drained, and mashed

1 (15-ounce) can corn kernels, drained

2 cups cooked polenta or ½ cup dry polenta

1 tablespoon Taco Seasoning (p. 98)

1 teaspoon salt

⅛ teaspoon pepper

Tortilla Chips (p. 100)

Heat olive oil in large saucepan over medium heat. Cook onions until soft and translucent. Add water or broth, tomatoes, black beans, mashed pinto beans, corn, polenta, Taco Seasoning, salt, and pepper. Heat to boiling. Reduce heat, and cook 30 minutes. Serve with Tortilla Chips.

Recipe Notes
• Substitute 1½ cups brown rice for polenta.
• Add a dollop of Guacamole with a Little Kick.
• Place corn in a food processor and pulse a few times for a creamy texture.
• Use kidney beans instead of black beans or pinto beans.

> Placing an onion briefly in the freezer before cutting it can reduce the amount of tear-shedding you experience. The sulphuric compound that makes your eyes water will not react as quickly when the onion is cold. However, don't freeze it for more than 8–10 minutes. (Too long will affect the taste.)

Tomato Basil Soup

½ tablespoon extra-virgin olive oil

½ cup chopped onion

3 (14.5-ounce) cans diced tomatoes, undrained

½ cup water

1 clove garlic, minced

1 teaspoon dried basil

1 teaspoon salt

⅛ teaspoon pepper

Toasted pumpkin seeds (pepitas) (optional for garnish)

Toasted raw sunflower seeds (optional for garnish)

YIELD: 4 servings
SERVING SIZE:
   about 1¼ cups

Heat olive oil in a large, deep skillet over medium heat. Add onions, and cook until soft and translucent. Add tomatoes, water, garlic, basil, salt, and pepper. Cook 20 minutes. Place mixture in a food processor or blender, and puree until desired consistency. (You may need to do this in two batches, because filling your processor or blender more than half full could cause the hot soup to pop the lid.) Return to skillet, and cook 5 – 10 more minutes. Garnish with toasted pumpkin and/or sunflower seeds, if desired.

Recipe Notes

• Substitute ½ cup chopped leeks for the onions (light green and white parts only).

> Although this recipe calls for canned tomatoes, you could easily use fresh, ripe tomatoes (peeled or unpeeled) instead. Put them in a food processor and puree until tomatoes reach the consistency you prefer.

Tuscan Soup

YIELD: 8 servings
SERVING SIZE:
about 1¼ cups

1 tablespoon extra-virgin olive oil

1 cup diced onion

1 cup diced carrots

2 cloves garlic, minced

6 cups water or Vegetable Broth (p. 134)

1 cup dry lentils, sorted and rinsed

1 (15-ounce) can cannellini beans, rinsed and drained

1 (14.5-ounce) can diced tomatoes, undrained

½ (10-ounce) package frozen chopped spinach, unthawed

½ tablespoon dried crushed rosemary

1 bay leaf

1 teaspoon salt

⅛ teaspoon pepper

Heat olive oil in large saucepan over medium heat. Add onions and carrots, and cook until onions are soft and translucent. Stir in garlic, and cook for 30 seconds, stirring constantly so garlic doesn't burn. Add water or broth, lentils, cannellini beans, tomatoes, spinach, rosemary, bay leaf, salt, and pepper. Heat to boiling, and then reduce heat. Simmer 20 – 25 minutes with lid tilted. Discard bay leaf before serving.

Recipe Notes
- Substitute chickpeas for cannellini beans.
- Add 1 cup cooked brown rice. (Add more broth or water if necessary.)
- Serve with Broiled Polenta Squares or Corn Muffins.
- To sort lentils, spread them in a single layer on an 11 by 17-inch baking sheet. Look for discolored and misshapen beans, and discard any unwanted particles. Place good lentils into a colander and rinse thoroughly using cold water.

> Lentils are tiny, disc-shaped legumes that are a top source of protein and fiber. They come in a range of colors, from brown and green to yellow and red. Lentils work well in soups, in salads, or as a side dish.

Vegetable Bean Soup

1 tablespoon extra-virgin olive oil

½ cup chopped onion

½ cup chopped carrots

½ cup chopped celery

1 clove garlic, minced

6 cups water

1 (8-ounce) can tomato sauce

1 (14.5-ounce) can light red kidney beans, rinsed and drained

1 (15-ounce) can black-eyed peas, rinsed and drained

1 (14.5-ounce) can French-style green beans, drained

1 cup chopped yellow summer squash, unpeeled

½ tablespoon chili powder

1 bay leaf

1 teaspoon salt

⅛ teaspoon pepper

2 tablespoons chopped fresh parsley

YIELD: 8 servings
SERVING SIZE:
    about 1¼ cups

Heat olive oil over medium heat in a large saucepan. Add onions, carrots, and celery. Cook until vegetables are softened. Add garlic, and cook for 30 seconds, stirring constantly so garlic doesn't burn. Pour in water and all remaining ingredients except parsley. Bring to a boil, and then lower heat. Simmer, uncovered, 30 minutes. Discard bay leaf and stir in parsley just before serving.

Recipe Notes

- Use 2 cups chopped fresh haricot vert beans instead of canned green beans. Haricot vert beans resemble regular green beans. However, they are a bit more slender and long, and they are also stringless. (A nice benefit!) When lightly cooked, haricot verts are tender, crispy, and very tasty, with a hint of sweetness.

> Homemade soups are a great way to get in your vegetable servings for the day.

Vegetable Broth

YIELD: 8 servings
SERVING SIZE:
about 1 cup

8   cups water
1   onion, quartered
2   carrots, unpeeled and cut into 2-inch chunks
2   celery stalks, cut into 2-inch chunks, leafy tops included
1   russet potato, unpeeled and cut into 2-inch chunks
4   white button mushrooms, sliced
⅛   cup fresh parsley or ½ tablespoon dried parsley
2   cloves garlic, peeled
1   bay leaf
1   teaspoon dried thyme
1   teaspoon salt
6   peppercorns

Place all ingredients in a large stockpot, and bring to a boil. Reduce heat, and simmer for about 45 minutes. Strain, cool, and refrigerate. Use as a base for soups.

Recipe Notes
- Experiment with other herbs and spices, such as basil, cumin, oregano, or red pepper flakes.
- Place strained vegetables in a food processor, and puree until smooth. Add to soups to thicken them.
- Other vegetables to use: leeks, parsnips, spinach, tomatoes, turnips, and/or zucchini.

> Bay leaves, which have a distinct fragrance and flavor, are a wonderful addition to any soup, sauce, or casserole. Fresh or dry leaves are most often used whole and discarded before serving.

Zucchini Soup

1½ pounds zucchini, peeled

2 tablespoons extra-virgin olive oil, divided

½ cup chopped onion

2 cloves garlic, minced

4 cups water

1 (15-ounce) can chickpeas, rinsed and drained

½ tablespoon dried basil

1 teaspoon salt

Toasted sunflower and/or pumpkin seeds (pepitas) for garnish

YIELD: 6 servings
SERVING SIZE:
   about 1 cup

Cut zucchini into 1-inch cubes, and set aside. Heat 1 tablespoon olive oil over medium heat in large saucepan. Add onions and garlic and cook until onions are soft and translucent. Add zucchini and stir in 1 tablespoon olive oil. Cook 3–5 minutes, stirring frequently. Pour in 4 cups water. Reduce heat and simmer 15 minutes.

Use a slotted spoon to remove zucchini and onions from the saucepan. Place them in a food processor or blender and process and until mixture is smooth. (You may need to do this in two batches, because filling your processor or blender more than half full could cause the hot soup to pop the lid.) Return pureed vegetables to saucepan.

Place chickpeas in food processor with about ½ cup of the soup from the saucepan and process until smooth. Add chickpea mixture to saucepan. Stir in basil and salt. Cook another 15 minutes. Serve with toasted sunflower and/or pumpkin seeds.

Recipe Notes

• For a chunkier soup with more texture, add another 15-ounce can chickpeas and leave whole.

• Use dried oregano flakes instead of basil.

• Double this recipe and freeze half of it for later use.

Zucchini is a type of summer squash that resembles a cucumber in shape and size. It has smooth, thin skin that is either green or yellow and can be striped or speckled. Its tender flesh is creamy white, and it contains numerous seeds.

Vegetables

Acorn Squash with Apples

1 pound acorn squash, unpeeled
3 cups sliced apples
2 cups unsweetened apple juice
¼ teaspoon cinnamon
¼ cup toasted chopped walnuts

YIELD: 4 servings
SERVING SIZE:
  about 1 cup

Preheat oven to 350 degrees. Cut squash crosswise into rings. Discard seeds and pulp. Place in a 9 by 13-inch baking dish. Distribute apples over squash. Mix cinnamon with apple juice, and pour over squash and apples. Bake 15 minutes. Flip squash and apples, and bake another 15 – 20 minutes. Remove squash from juice, and peel skin. Cut each ring into 1-inch cubes. To serve, place about ½ cup squash, ½ cup apples, and 1 tablespoon apple juice in each bowl. Top with 1 tablespoon walnuts.

Recipe Notes
- Mix the remaining apple juice in with oatmeal, or use to make Apple-Cinnamon Salad Dressing.
- Substitute chopped almonds or pecans for the walnuts.
- Sprinkle unsweetened coconut flakes over all.

When selecting acorn squash, choose squash that is firm and heavy for its size, without any soft spots or cracks. Store in a cool, dry place away from extreme temperatures and sunlight. Ideally, squash should be refrigerated only once it has been cut or cooked, as it will suffer damage at temperatures below 50 degrees.

Artichoke Tomato Sauce

1 (14-ounce) can artichoke hearts, ¼ cup juice reserved
1 tablespoon extra-virgin olive oil
1 cup chopped onion
2 cloves garlic, minced
3 (14.5-ounce) cans diced tomatoes, undrained
½ tablespoon dried basil
½ tablespoon dried parsley

YIELD: 12 servings
SERVING SIZE:
  about ½ cup

Vegetables

1 teaspoon dried oregano flakes

¼ teaspoon salt

Pinch cayenne pepper

Put artichokes in a food processor, and pulse just long enough to break into smaller pieces. Set aside. Heat olive oil in a large saucepan or stockpot, and cook onions until soft and translucent. Add garlic, and cook for 30 seconds, stirring constantly so garlic doesn't burn. Add tomatoes, artichokes, reserved artichoke juice, basil, parsley, oregano, salt, and cayenne pepper. Bring to a boil, and then lower heat. Simmer 30 minutes.

Recipe Notes

• Serve with brown rice, lentils, quinoa, spaghetti squash, or whole grain pasta.

• Add chopped kale, mushrooms, or spinach.

• Top with chopped black olives.

Buying a fresh artichoke can be intimidating. Its pokey leaves look like they could leave a nasty cut! However, if you are brave enough to tackle this funny-looking vegetable, the reward is the tasty, tender artichoke heart. The heart of the artichoke is the fleshy center section that is most suitable for eating. To prepare an artichoke, rinse well under cold running water. Peel off the hard outer petals. Cut about 1 inch off the pointed top, and cut off the bottom stem. Trim tips of leaves with scissors, if desired. (Some people like the look of clipped petals, but it really isn't necessary to remove the thorns, because they soften with cooking.) Dip or rub with lemon juice to preserve color.

Asparagus-Mushroom Sauté

YIELD: 8 servings
SERVING SIZE:
about ½ cup

1 tablespoon extra-virgin olive oil

1 cup thinly sliced onion, sliced pole to pole (see Recipe Notes)

3 cups sliced white button mushrooms

1 pound asparagus spears, trimmed and cut into 1-inch pieces

2 cloves garlic, minced

1½ teasoons dried oregano flakes

½ teaspoon salt

⅛ teaspoon pepper

Heat olive oil over medium heat in a large skillet. Add onions, mushrooms, asparagus, garlic, oregano, salt, and pepper. Increase heat to medium-high, and cook 5 – 7 minutes or until vegetables are crisp tender, stirring frequently.

Recipe Notes

- To slice an onion pole to pole, or into half rings, think of the onion as a globe. Trim root end (south pole) and stem end (north pole). Peel off outer layers. Cut onion in half from north pole to south pole, making a series of vertical slices perpendicular to the equator of the onion.
- Add chickpeas and brown rice to make this sauté a main dish.
- Use as a topping for Mashed Potato and Corn Casserole or a baked potato.
- Serve with lentils or quinoa.

> *Sauté* is French for "to jump," which describes the method of cooking in which food is cooked quickly in a small amount of butter or oil. The food "jumps" as it is either rapidly stirred or shaken over the heat.

Baked Potato Chips

2 pounds russet baking potatoes, peeled

1 tablespoon extra-virgin olive oil

½ teaspoon salt

⅛ teaspoon pepper

YIELD: 4 servings
SERVING SIZE:
  about 1 cup

Preheat oven to 375 degrees. Cut potatoes into thin ⅛-inch discs with the slicing disc of a food processor, with a mandolin slicer, or by hand. Place potato slices in a large bowl. Add olive oil, salt, and pepper, and stir well to coat. Spread in a single layer on two large 11 by 17-inch baking sheets. Bake 15 minutes. Flip potatoes, and cook another 10 – 15 minutes, or until chips are crispy.

Recipe Notes

- Thin chips will be done earlier than thicker ones, so remove them from the oven so that they don't burn and continue cooking the thick chips until done.
- Add garlic powder and/or rosemary.
- Use sweet potatoes instead of russet potatoes. (They won't get as crispy due to their higher water content.)

> Baked potatoes are loaded with vitamin B6, which plays an important role in the proper functioning of the nervous system. Vitamin B6 is also necessary for the breakdown of glycogen, the form in which sugar is stored in our muscle cells and liver, so this vitamin is a key player in athletic performance and endurance.

Classic Tomato Sauce

YIELD: 8 servings
SERVING SIZE:
about ½ cup

1 tablespoon extra-virgin olive oil
½ cup chopped onion
2 cloves garlic, minced
1 (29-ounce) can tomato puree
1 (6-ounce) can tomato paste
½ cup water
1 bay leaf
1 teaspoon dried basil
1 teaspoon dried parsley
½ teaspoon salt
⅛ teaspoon pepper

Heat olive oil in a large skillet, and add onions. Cook until soft and translucent. Stir in garlic, and cook 30 seconds, stirring constantly so garlic doesn't burn. Add remaining ingredients, and cook, uncovered, over low heat for 30 minutes. Discard bay leaf before serving.

Recipe Notes

- Substitute a can of crushed tomatoes for the tomato puree.
- Add diced green bell peppers, sliced mushrooms, or black olives.

- Pour over Pan-Roasted Broccoli and Cauliflower.
- Serve with Lentil-Spinach "Meatballs" and brown rice, spaghetti squash, or whole grain pasta.
- When tomatoes are in season, use 3 – 4 fresh, ripe tomatoes (peeled, seeded, and cored) instead of canned. Puree in food processor or blender until smooth.

> While it may be more convenient to pick up a jar of tomato sauce at the store, you can't beat the taste of homemade. All you need is a few ingredients and a little bit of time, and the result is well worth it.

Delicata Squash Rings

2 delicata squash (about 1½ to 2 pounds), unpeeled
1 tablespoon extra-virgin olive oil
½ teaspoon dried parsley
¼ teaspoon dried thyme
¼ teaspoon salt
⅛ teaspoon pepper

YIELD: 4 servings
SERVING SIZE:
   about 5 – 6 rings

Preheat oven to 425 degrees. Cut squash into ½-inch rings. Scoop out seeds and pulp from the middle of each ring and discard. (A small ice-cream scoop works well.) Lightly rub an 11 by 17-inch baking sheet with olive oil, and place rings on sheet. Do not overlap. Place olive oil, parsley, thyme, salt, and pepper in a large bowl. Mix in squash, and stir well to coat. Bake 15 minutes. Flip, and bake 10 minutes more or until golden brown and tender.

Recipe Notes
- Instead of delicata squash, you can use butternut squash. Peel squash and cut into wedges or cubes before baking.

> Delicata squash, also known as peanut squash or sweet potato squash, is an oblong squash that has a cream-colored, green-striped skin. It tastes mild and fairly sweet, and has a nice, buttery texture, similar to that of sweet potatoes.

Vegetables

Dillicious Peas and Carrots

YIELD: 4 servings
SERVING SIZE:
   about ½ cup

1   tablespoon extra-virgin olive oil

½   cup chopped onion

1   clove garlic, minced

1   cup cooked chopped carrots

1   cup cooked sweet peas

½   teaspoon salt

¼   teaspoon dried dill

Heat olive oil in skillet over medium heat. Add onions, and cook until soft and translucent. Stir in garlic, carrots, and peas. Add salt and dill, and cook until heated through. Serve immediately.

We've been told since childhood how good carrots are for us. They are an excellent source of beta-carotene and antioxidant compounds, which help protect against cardiovascular disease and cancer and also promote good vision. Many people, though, don't realize that peas are packed with nutrition as well. Although they are tiny, peas contain eight vitamins, seven minerals, dietary fiber, and protein.

Eggplant Tomato Sauce

YIELD: 12 servings
SERVING SIZE:
   about ½ cup

1½   pounds eggplant, peeled, cut into 1-inch cubes

1   tablespoon salt

1   tablespoon extra-virgin olive oil, divided

½   cup diced onion

1   clove garlic, minced

1   (28-ounce) can crushed tomatoes

1   (14.5-ounce) can diced tomatoes, undrained

2   tablespoons chopped fresh parsley

2   teaspoons dried basil

1   teaspoon dried oregano flakes

1   bay leaf

⅛   teaspoon pepper

Preheat oven to 350 degrees. Place eggplant cubes in a large colander in the sink, and sprinkle with salt. Use your hands to toss eggplant so that cubes are well coated. Let drain 30 minutes. In a large saucepan, heat ½ tablespoon olive oil over medium heat. Cook onions 3 – 5 minutes or until soft and translucent. Add garlic, and cook for 30 seconds, stirring constantly so garlic doesn't burn. Add crushed and diced tomatoes, parsley, basil, oregano, bay leaf, and pepper. Simmer, covered, for 30 minutes over low heat.

Pat eggplant dry with paper towels. Heat a large skillet with ½ tablespoon olive oil, and cook eggplant 3 – 5 minutes, stirring constantly. (You may have to do this in two batches if you don't have a skillet large enough to do all at once.) Once eggplant is slightly browned, place it in a 9 by 13-inch baking dish that has been rubbed with olive oil. Discard bay leaf from tomato mixture, and pour over eggplant. Bake uncovered for 30 minutes.

Recipe Notes
- Use as a sauce with brown rice, lentils, spaghetti squash, or whole grain pasta.
- Top with black olives.
- Add chopped kale or spinach to sauce.
- For a smoother sauce, put in food processor or blender until desired consistency is reached.
- Substitute 2 (14.5-ounce) cans diced tomatoes for the crushed tomatoes.

Eggplant is a member of the nightshade family of vegetables, which also includes tomatoes, sweet peppers, and potatoes. Its skin is a glossy deep purple, and the flesh is cream-colored with a pleasantly bitter taste. The spongy texture of the eggplant gives it a meaty taste.

Garlic Spring Peas with Leeks

  3 cups water
  1 pound fresh or frozen spring peas
  1 tablespoon extra-virgin olive oil
  ½ cup chopped leeks (light green and white parts only)

YIELD: 6 servings
SERVING SIZE:
  about ½ cup

2 cloves garlic, minced

½ teaspoon salt

⅛ teaspoon pepper

On stovetop, heat water in medium saucepan to boiling. Place peas in boiling water, and cover. Bring to a second boil. Reduce heat, and simmer 6 – 8 minutes. While peas are cooking, heat olive oil in a small skillet over medium heat. Add leeks and garlic, and cook 3 – 5 minutes, stirring constantly. Drain peas, and stir in leeks, salt, and pepper.

Recipe Notes
- Use diced onions instead of leeks.
- Add basil or oregano.
- Steam the peas for 8 – 10 minutes instead of boiling them.

> Leeks, which look like giant, overgrown scallions, are related to the onion family but have a sweeter taste. They have a long, cylindrical stalk with a very small white bulb. When selecting leeks, look for slender, straight ones. The top green leaves should look fresh. Avoid leeks with wilted or yellowing tops.

Ginger-Garlic Baby Carrots

YIELD: 6 servings
SERVING SIZE:
about ½ cup

1 pound baby carrots or 1 pound carrots, peeled and cut into 2-inch pieces

½ tablespoon extra-virgin olive oil

2 tablespoons minced onion

1 clove garlic, minced

½ teaspoon minced fresh ginger root or ⅛ teaspoon dried ginger

⅛ teaspoon salt

Grated ginger root

Boil or steam carrots until crisp tender (15 – 20 minutes). While carrots are cooking, heat olive oil over medium heat in a small skillet. Add onions, and cook until soft and translucent. Stir in garlic and ginger root. Cook for 30 seconds, stirring constantly so garlic doesn't burn. Add carrots and salt, and stir well to coat. Transfer to a serving dish, and grate a little fresh ginger root on top.

Ginger is the gnarled, bumpy root of the ginger plant. Its flavor is peppery and slightly sweet. Ginger root has a very thin, light brown skin that must be removed before using. Simply cut off the amount of ginger you need, and use a paring knife or vegetable peeler to remove the skin. Fresh, unpeeled ginger root should be wrapped in paper towels, placed in a plastic bag, and refrigerated up to three weeks. It can also be tightly wrapped in plastic and frozen up to two months.

Green Beans with Rays of Sunshine

1 pound fresh or frozen green beans
1 yellow bell pepper, seeded and cored
½ tablespoon extra-virgin olive oil
¼ cup minced onion
½ teaspoon dried dill
½ teaspoon salt
⅛ teaspoon pepper

YIELD: 6 servings
SERVING SIZE:
about ½ cup

Steam green beans 20 – 22 minutes or until crisp tender (or boil in a large saucepan about 8 – 10 minutes). While green beans are cooking, grate yellow pepper in a food processor (use shredder attachment) or by hand. Drain any liquid, and set aside.

When green beans are done cooking, heat olive oil in a large skillet over medium heat. Add onions and yellow pepper. Cook until onions are soft and translucent. Add green beans, dill, salt, and pepper. Stir well, and serve immediately.

The inspiration for this recipe came one March evening, when the weather was turning warmer, and I had a bad case of spring fever. As I prepared green beans for dinner, I decided to add a little springlike touch instead of serving them plain. My husband took one look at my new concoction and immediately named them Green Beans with Rays of Sunshine.

Vegetables

Green Beans with Toasted Walnuts

YIELD: 6 servings
SERVING SIZE:
about ½ cup

1 pound fresh or frozen green beans
½ tablespoon extra-virgin olive oil
½ teaspoon salt
¼ teaspoon tarragon
⅛ teaspoon pepper
2 tablespoons finely diced toasted walnuts

Wash fresh beans thoroughly and trim ends. Cut into bite-size pieces. If using a steamer, cook 20 – 22 minutes. If boiling, cover the beans with cold water in a large saucepan, and bring to a boil. Reduce heat, and simmer until crisp tender, about 8 – 10 minutes. Drain green beans, and stir in olive oil, salt, tarragon, pepper, and walnuts. Serve immediately.

Recipe Notes
• Substitute pecans for walnuts.

> Walnuts are unique compared to other nuts because they're the only type of nut with a significant amount of alpha-linolenic acid, the plant-based source of omega-3 fatty acids. Omega-3 fatty acids help to reduce inflammation in the body, promote healthy cell membranes, and help prevent cancer growth.

Grilled Veggie Kebabs

YIELD: 8 servings
SERVING SIZE: 1 skewer

Marinade
2 tablespoons extra-virgin olive oil
2 tablespoons lemon juice or pineapple juice
1 tablespoon Bragg's Liquid Aminos or soy sauce
1 clove garlic, minced
¼ teaspoon ground ginger

Vegetables
16 cherry tomatoes
16 white button mushrooms, stems removed
1 red or green bell pepper, cut into 2-inch pieces (about 1 cup)
1 yellow or orange bell pepper, cut into 2-inch pieces (about 1 cup)

1 cup chopped onion, cut into 2-inch pieces

1 cup zucchini, cut into 2-inch pieces

8 (10-inch) metal or wooden skewers (soak wooden ones in water for 15 minutes before using so that they don't burn)

Prepare marinade in small bowl, and set aside.

Place vegetables on skewers, alternating as you go. Set skewers in a 9 by 13-inch casserole dish, and brush vegetables with marinade. Cover, and let sit at room temperature 30 minutes. If you have any remaining marinade, reserve it to coat vegetables while cooking.

Preheat grill. Place skewers over medium heat and grill 10 minutes or until done, turning occasionally as needed.

Recipe Notes

• Use Italian Salad Dressing or Orange – Poppy Seed Salad Dressing as a marinade.
• Other vegetable ideas are cucumbers, olives, potatoes, or yellow squash.

> If using an indoor grill, you don't need to soak the skewers.

Italian-Style Broccoli

2 – 3 broccoli crowns, cut into florets with 1-inch stems (about 6 cups)

1 tablespoon extra-virgin olive oil

2 cups halved cherry tomatoes

1 cup chopped fennel bulb

½ cup chopped onion

1 clove garlic, minced

2 tablespoons chopped fresh basil or 1½ teaspoons dried basil

2 tablespoons pine nuts, toasted

YIELD: 6 servings
SERVING SIZE:
about 1 cup

Steam broccoli 10 – 12 minutes, or boil 5 – 7 minutes. Set aside. Heat oil in large skillet over medium heat. Add tomatoes, fennel, onion, garlic, and basil. Cook about 10 minutes, stirring frequently. Just before serving, stir in broccoli and pine nuts. Cook until heated through, and serve.

Recipe Notes

• Substitute chopped cucumbers or zucchini for the fennel.

> Broccoli is one of the most nutritious vegetables you can eat. It contains vitamin C, vitamin A (mostly as beta-carotene), folic acid, calcium, and fiber. Broccoli is also a rich source of a variety of biochemicals that are known to fight cancer.

Kale with Tomatoes and Onions

YIELD: 6 servings
SERVING SIZE:
about ½ cup

4 ounces curly kale, stems removed and coarsely chopped (about 6 cups)
1 tablespoon extra-virgin olive oil
1 cup thinly sliced onion, sliced pole to pole (see Recipe Notes)
2 cloves garlic, minced
3 cups chopped tomatoes, unpeeled, unseeded
1 teaspoon dried basil
1 teaspoon dried oregano flakes
½ teaspoon salt
Pine nuts (optional)

In a large skillet, heat olive oil over medium heat. Add onions and garlic. Put tomatoes in a large bowl, and squeeze with your hands so that some juice is extracted. Pour tomatoes with their juice into skillet with onions and garlic, and cook 15 minutes. Stir in kale, basil, oregano, and salt. Cover, and simmer 5 – 7 minutes, or until the kale has softened. Sprinkle pine nuts on top, if desired. Serve immediately.

Recipe Notes

• To slice an onion pole to pole, or into half rings, think of the onion as a globe. Trim root end (south pole) and stem end (north pole). Peel off outer layers. Cut onion in half from north pole to south pole, making a series of vertical slices perpendicular to the equator of the onion.
• Serve over cooked brown or wild rice, lentils, or quinoa.
• Add ½ cup cannellini beans or chickpeas.
• Use fresh spinach leaves instead of kale.

Kale is a leafy green member of the cabbage family of vegetables, along with broccoli, Brussels sprouts, cauliflower, and turnips. The different varieties are curly kale, ornamental kale, and dinosaur kale, all of which differ in taste, texture, and appearance.

Curly kale has ruffled leaves and a fibrous stalk and is usually deep green in color. It has a pungent taste with a bitter peppery flavor. Ornamental kale leaves may be green, white, or purple, and have a mild flavor and a tender texture. Dinosaur kale, or lacinato kale, features dark blue-green leaves that have a sweeter and more delicate taste than curly kale.

Lima Beans with Thyme

2 cups frozen lima beans
½ tablespoon extra-virgin olive oil
¼ cup chopped onion
2 tablespoons chopped fresh parsley
½ teaspoon salt
¼ teaspoon dried thyme

YIELD: 4 servings
SERVING SIZE:
about ½ cup

Cook lima beans on stovetop according to package directions. While beans are cooking, heat olive oil in a small skillet over medium heat. Add onions, and cook until soft and translucent. Drain beans, and mix in onion. Add parsley, salt, and thyme. Stir well, and serve.

Recipe Notes
• Add 1 (14.5-ounce) can of drained corn kernels.
• Served chilled as a salad topping.

Lima beans are a good source of fiber. The benefits of fiber in the diet are numerous—promotes health, lowers cholesterol, helps reduce the risk of some chronic diseases, prevents constipation, and helps control blood sugar levels.

Marinated Zucchini

YIELD: 8 servings
SERVING SIZE:
  about ½ cup

2 pounds zucchini, unpeeled
1½ tablespoons olive oil
1 clove garlic, minced
1½ teaspoons dried oregano flakes
½ teaspoon salt
⅛ teaspoon pepper
1 teaspoon fresh lemon juice

Preheat oven to 475 degrees. Trim ends of zucchini, and cut in half lengthwise. Feed zucchini halves through the tube of a food processor with the slicing disc attached. You may also use a mandolin slicer to cut the zucchini into thin slices, or cut them by hand. Place slices in a large bowl. Add olive oil, and stir to coat. Mix in garlic, oregano, salt, and pepper. Stir again.

Place zucchini on two large 11 by 17-inch baking sheets, trying to separate the pieces as much as possible so they are in a single layer. Roast 10 minutes, flip, and then roast another 5 minutes. Edges of zucchini should be slightly browned and crispy.

Remove zucchini from oven, and put in a large dish. Stir in lemon juice. Cover, and let sit at least 1 – 2 hours. Serve at room temperature.

Recipe Notes
• Use as the base for Marinated Vegetable Salad.
• Sprinkle with pine nuts before serving.
• Substitute yellow summer squash for half of the zucchini.

Marinated Zucchini is the recipe that inspired the creation of my blog, which eventually led to the publication of this book. You can see why it's one of my favorites.

Mashed Potato and Corn Casserole

2 pounds russet potatoes, peeled and cubed

¼ cup unsweetened almond milk or soy milk

1 (14.5-ounce) can corn kernels, drained

2 tablespoons chopped fresh parsley

1 teaspoon salt

⅛ teaspoon pepper

½ tablespoon extra-virgin olive oil

½ cup diced onion

½ cup chopped green onion (green parts only)

2 cloves garlic, minced

Topping

¼ cup yellow cornmeal

½ tablespoon extra-virgin olive oil

½ teaspoon garlic powder

Boil or steam potatoes until tender (about 20 minutes). Pour in almond milk, and mash until smooth. Put corn in a food processor and process about 10 seconds. Mix corn with potatoes, and add parsley, salt, and pepper.

Preheat oven to 350 degrees. Heat olive oil over medium heat, and cook onions and green onions until soft and translucent. Add garlic, and cook 30 seconds, stirring constantly so garlic doesn't burn. Stir into potato-corn mixture, and mix well. Lightly rub a 9 by 13-inch casserole dish with olive oil, and spread mixture into dish. In a small bowl, use a fork to mix cornmeal, olive oil, and garlic powder until well blended. Sprinkle over top of casserole, and bake 30 minutes.

Potatoes contain more potassium than any other vegetable and even more than a banana. One serving of a 5-ounce potato with the skin on has 720 mg, more than the following high potassium foods: broccoli (540 mg per serving), bananas (400 mg per serving), tomatoes (360 mg per serving), and oranges (260 mg per serving). Potassium is necessary for body growth, cell maintenance, nerve function, and for normal muscle contraction, including the heart muscle.

Recipe Notes

- Substitute 1 – 2 tablespoons fresh chives or ½ tablespoon dried chives for the green onions.
- Stir in 1 cup of steamed chopped broccoli.
- Top with sliced olives.
- Add 1 (4-ounce) can of chopped green chilies, drained.

Vegetables

Pan-Roasted Broccoli and Cauliflower

YIELD: 8 servings

SERVING SIZE:
about 1 cup

1 tablespoon extra-virgin olive oil

½ cup diced onion

3 cups broccoli florets

3 cups cauliflower florets

1 tablespoon fresh oregano or 1 teaspoon dried oregano flakes

½ teaspoon salt

Heat olive oil in a large, deep skillet over medium heat. Add onion and cook 3 – 5 minutes or until soft and translucent. Stir in broccoli and cauliflower. Turn vegetables a few times to coat with the olive oil. Sprinkle in oregano and salt. Cover, and cook 7 – 8 minutes, stirring frequently. Vegetables should be slightly browned and crisp tender when ready to serve.

Recipe Notes
• Top with Classic Tomato Sauce.
• Add one clove of minced garlic.
• Use basil instead of oregano.

Broccoli is an excellent source of vitamin C and calcium. One-half cup of cooked, chopped broccoli provides the same amount of vitamin C as ½ cup of orange juice. Broccoli's dark green color indicates that it is a good source of vitamin A. Cauliflower is also high in vitamin C and is a good source of potassium. By combining these superfoods, you have an extremely nutrient-rich vegetable dish.

Pesto Spaghetti Squash

YIELD: 6 servings

SERVING SIZE:
about ½ cup

2 pounds spaghetti squash

1 recipe Pesto (p. 94)

Preheat oven to 375 degrees. With a fork, prick squash all over and place in baking dish. Cook 1 hour, and remove from oven.

Let squash cool 10 – 15 minutes before cutting in half and removing the seeds. Discard seeds. Pull a fork lengthwise through the flesh to separate it into long strands. Place strands in a large bowl.

Add enough Pesto to coat spaghetti squash strands. Mix well, and serve immediately.

Recipe Notes

- Substitute whole grain pasta for the spaghetti squash.
- If Pesto has been refrigerated, be sure to rewarm before adding to spaghetti squash for easier mixing.

> Spaghetti squash is a fabulous food. In my opinion, it's one of the most unique vegetables God made. After it has been cooked, the flesh of the squash comes out like thin spaghetti strands. Every time I eat one, I'm reminded of just how creative our God is.

Roasted Root Vegetables

1 pound parsnips, peeled and cut into 1-inch pieces
1 pound rutabaga, peeled and cut into 1-inch pieces
1 pound sweet potatoes, peeled and cut into 1-inch pieces
1½ tablespoons extra-virgin olive oil
½ teaspoon salt
⅛ teaspoon pepper

YIELD: 8 servings
SERVING SIZE:
about 1 cup

Preheat oven to 400 degrees. Combine vegetables in a large bowl, and add olive oil, salt, and pepper. Stir well to coat. Spread out on two 11 by 17-inch baking sheets, making sure the pieces don't overlap. Roast 15 minutes, stir, and return to oven. Roast 15 minutes more. You may serve vegetables at this point if you want them crispy on the outside but slightly soft on the inside. Cook for another 15 minutes if you like a crunchier texture.

Recipe Notes

- Try a different vegetable combination, such as carrots, red potatoes, and turnips.

> Root vegetables are the underground parts of plants that are eaten as vegetables. Carrots, garlic, onions, parsnips, potatoes, rutabagas, and turnips are all root vegetables.

Rockin' Rosemary Turnips

YIELD: 4 servings
SERVING SIZE:
about ½ cup

1 tablespoon extra-virgin olive oil

1 cup thinly sliced onion, sliced pole to pole (see Recipe Notes)

1 pound turnips, peeled and quartered

1 clove garlic, minced

½ teaspoon dried crushed rosemary, divided

½ teaspoon salt

⅛ teaspoon pepper

Heat olive oil in large skillet over medium-low heat. Add onions and stir to coat with olive oil. Cook 15 minutes, or until slightly browned. While onions are cooking, boil or steam turnips for 20 minutes or until tender. Mash until smooth (like mashed potatoes), and stir in ¼ teaspoon rosemary, salt, and pepper. Keep warm until ready to serve. Add garlic and the other ¼ teaspoon rosemary to onions in skillet. Cook 1 – 2 minutes, and serve with mashed turnips.

Recipe Notes

- Substitute russet potatoes for turnips.
- To slice an onion pole to pole, or into half rings, think of the onion as a globe. Trim root end (south pole) and stem end (north pole). Peel off outer layers. Cut onion in half from north pole to south pole, making a series of vertical slices perpendicular to the equator of the onion.

Turnips are root vegetables that are about the size of an apple. They have firm white skin with bright purple around the top part, which has been exposed to the sun. When buying turnips, always choose smaller ones for a sweeter flavor. Larger turnips tend to have a woodier texture. Look for turnips that have a smooth skin and are free of blemishes. Store in the refrigerator crisper, and use within a week or so.

Rosemary Red Potatoes

2 pounds B-size new red potatoes (about 10 – 12 total)
1 tablespoon extra-virgin olive oil
½ teaspoon dried crushed rosemary
½ teaspoon salt
⅛ teaspoon pepper

YIELD: 4 servings
SERVING SIZE:
about ½ cup

Scrub potatoes well. Place in large saucepan, and cover with water. Heat to boiling. Reduce heat, and simmer 15 minutes. Drain, and allow to cool slightly.

Preheat oven to 425 degrees. Cut potatoes into quarters, and return to saucepan. Add olive oil, rosemary, salt, and pepper. Stir to coat. Place potatoes on an 11 by 17-inch baking sheet. Bake 30 minutes, turning potatoes about halfway through cooking time.

Recipe Notes
• Add sliced or quartered onions.
• Use turnips (peeled, quartered) instead of red potatoes.

New red potatoes range from the size of a golf ball to the size of a baseball. They are graded as A or B, with the B-size potato being the smaller of the two.

Sweet Potato Pie

2 pounds sweet potatoes
½ cup Date Honey (p. 87)
¼ cup unsweetened orange juice
1 cup oat flour (see Recipe Notes)
1 teaspoon grated orange zest
½ teaspoon cinnamon
⅛ teaspoon nutmeg
¼ cup unsweetened coconut flakes
¼ cup finely chopped pecans

YIELD: 8 servings
SERVING SIZE:
about 1 slice pie

Vegetables

Preheat oven to 350 degrees. Bake or steam sweet potatoes until tender. If baking, pierce each potato a few times with a fork and wrap tightly in aluminum foil, shiny side out. Bake at least 1 hour or until soft. Remove from oven, and set aside until cool enough to handle. Peel and discard skins. If steaming, peel skins and cook 25 – 30 minutes or according to your steamer's directions. Cut potatoes into smaller pieces, and mash with a potato masher.

Put potatoes, Date Honey, and orange juice in a food processor or blender, and puree until completely smooth with no lumps. Add oat flour, orange zest, cinnamon, and nutmeg. Stir well.

Pour sweet potato mixture into a 9 by 2-inch pie plate that has been rubbed with olive oil. Spread coconut flakes and pecans over top. Bake 15 – 20 minutes, or until lightly browned. Serve immediately.

Recipe Notes
- Spread almond butter or Date Honey on top of each serving.
- Add ½ cup raisins when you mix the oats and pureed potato mixture.
- Substitute walnuts for the pecans.
- Make your own oat flour by placing old-fashioned rolled oats in a food processor or blender until fine. (1 cup old-fashioned oats will yield about ¾ cup ground oats.)
- The zest is the outermost, colorful skin of citrus fruits. Zest is often used to enhance flavor in recipes. The pith, or white membrane underneath the outside peel, has a bitter, unpleasant taste and should be avoided while zesting.

> Eating sweet potatoes is like having dessert. This recipe combines them with other naturally sweet foods — cinnamon, coconut, dates, and oranges — for a wonderfully tasty (and healthy!) pie.

Tarragon Roasted Asparagus

1   pound asparagus spears, trimmed (36 – 40 thin spears or 18 – 20 thick spears)
½   tablespoon extra-virgin olive oil
½   teaspoon dried tarragon
½   teaspoon garlic powder
¼   teaspoon salt

YIELD: 6 servings
SERVING SIZE: about
6 – 7 thin spears or
3 – 4 thick spears

Preheat oven to 450 degrees. Lightly rub an 11 by 17-inch baking sheet with olive oil, and place asparagus spears on sheet in one layer. Brush asparagus with olive oil. Combine tarragon, garlic powder, and salt in a small bowl. Sprinkle over spears, and then roll to coat. Roast 15 minutes.

Recipe Notes
• Substitute basil, oregano, or rosemary for the tarragon.

Not all asparagus spears are created equal. You will typically find two kinds: thin-stemmed spears and thick spears. The thin spears are younger and haven't reached maturity. Since they are still growing, the spears will contain a greater amount of fiber, making their texture tougher and chewier than the larger, thicker ones. I have used both kinds in this recipe and usually prefer the thick stems so I don't have to work as hard to enjoy them! Use asparagus within a day or two after purchasing for best flavor. Store in the refrigerator with the ends wrapped in a damp paper towel.

Vegetables

Yukon Vegetable Bake

YIELD: 4 servings
SERVING SIZE:
about 1 cup

1 pound Yukon Gold potatoes, unpeeled and cut into ½-inch cubes
1 cup fresh corn kernels (about 2 ears)
2 tablespoons extra-virgin olive oil, divided
½ teaspoon salt
¼ teaspoon dried basil
⅛ teaspoon pepper
1 cup thinly sliced onion, sliced pole to pole
2 cups chopped zucchini, unpeeled, cut into ¼-inch rounds
2 cloves garlic, minced

Preheat oven to 425 degrees. Mix potatoes and corn in a large bowl. Add 1 tablespoon olive oil, salt, basil, and pepper. Stir well. Place on an 11 by 17-inch baking sheet. Bake about 25 minutes, stirring halfway through cooking time.

When potatoes have about 5 minutes of cooking time remaining, heat 1 tablespoon olive oil in a large skillet over medium heat. Add onions and zucchini. Cook until vegetables are slightly browned. Stir in garlic, and cook about 30 seconds, stirring constantly so garlic doesn't burn. Add potatoes and corn. Stir well, and cook another 5 minutes before serving.

Recipe Notes
• Use yellow crookneck squash instead of zucchini.
• To slice an onion pole to pole, or into half rings, think of the onion as a globe. Trim root end (south pole) and stem end (north pole). Peel off outer layers. Cut onion in half from north pole to south pole, making a series of vertical slices perpendicular to the equator of the onion.

Yukon Gold potatoes are slightly flat and oval in shape with light gold, thin skin and light yellow flesh. Developed in Canada, they are a cross between a North American white potato and a wild South American yellow-fleshed one. Yukon Golds have a higher sugar content than russet potatoes, which results in their buttery flavor and moist flesh.

Main Dishes

Main Dishes

Antipasto Pizza Pie

YIELD: 4 – 6 servings
SERVING SIZE:
 1 – 2 slices pie

Crust

    3   cups cooked brown rice
    2   tablespoons extra-virgin olive oil
    ¼   cup oat flour (see Recipe Notes)
    ¼   teaspoon garlic powder
    ¼   teaspoon onion powder

Sauce

    1   (8-ounce) can tomato sauce
    1   teaspoon dried basil
    1   teaspoon dried oregano flakes
    1   teaspoon dried parsley
    ¼   teaspoon garlic powder

Toppings

    ¼   cup chopped canned artichokes, drained
    ¼   cup chopped black olives
    ¼   cup chopped jarred roasted red bell peppers, drained
    2   ounces extra-firm tofu, grated (about ½ cup)
    1   tablespoon chopped fresh parsley

Recipe Notes

- Make your own oat flour by placing old-fashioned rolled oats in a food processor or blender and process until fine (1 cup old-fashioned oats will yield about ¾ cup ground oats).
- If you don't have a grater, use your hands to crumble tofu into small pieces.
- Other topping ideas are diced green peppers, mushrooms, onions, spinach, and zucchini.

Preheat oven to 400 degrees. Mix rice, olive oil, oat flour, garlic powder, and onion powder in a large bowl. Stir well. Rub bottom and sides of a 9 by 2-inch pie plate with olive oil. Press rice evenly over bottom and up about 1 inch along sides to make the crust. Bake 8 – 10 minutes or until rice is lightly browned. Combine tomato sauce, basil, oregano, parsley, and garlic powder in a small bowl. Spread over crust, and top with artichokes, olives, and peppers. Sprinkle grated tofu and parsley over all. Bake 10 minutes. Let pie rest 5 minutes so slices stay intact when you serve them.

Antipasto is an Italian word meaning "before the pasta." Antipasto is the traditional first course of a formal Italian meal. Typically, it is an assortment of cold hors d'oeuvres that includes meats, olives, cheese, and vegetables.

Black Bean Chili Bake

2 (15-ounce) cans black beans, rinsed and drained

2 (8-ounce) cans tomato sauce

2 cups cooked brown rice

1 (14.5-ounce) can corn kernels, drained

1 cup chopped jarred roasted red bell peppers, drained (see Recipe Notes)

½ cup diced onion

1 tablespoon chili powder

YIELD: 6 servings
SERVING SIZE:
   about 1 cup

Preheat oven to 350 degrees. Put beans in a large bowl, and mash until they're about half crushed. Add tomato sauce, rice, corn, peppers, onion, and chili powder. Stir to combine. Rub a 9 by 13-inch casserole dish with olive oil, and place mixture in it. Bake 20 minutes, or until heated through.

Recipe Notes

- Serve alone or as a filling for Whole Grain Tortillas.
- Use as a dip with Tortilla Chips.
- Spread on top of Broiled Polenta Squares.
- Another option is to boil the peppers instead of roasting them. Simply remove stems and seeds, and cut into pieces. Place in boiling water, and cook for 5 minutes.
- Additional topping ideas include avocado slices, cherry tomatoes, green onions, and/or black olives.

To roast your own peppers, cut them in halves or quarters. Remove seeds and membranes, and put peppers on an 11 by 17-inch baking sheet, skin side up. Place the baking sheet on a rack in the oven about 4 inches from the broiling unit. Broil 20 minutes, or until skins are browned.

Immediately transfer the peppers to a paper or plastic bag. Seal, and let stand 20 minutes. The steam within the bag will help to loosen the skins. Remove from the bag. When cool enough to handle, remove peel with hands or a knife.

Main Dishes

Caribbean Wild Rice

YIELD: 6 servings
SERVING SIZE:
about 1 cup

1 tablespoon extra-virgin olive oil
½ cup chopped onion
1 clove garlic, minced
1 (8-ounce) can unsweetened pineapple tidbits, juice reserved
2 tablespoons Bragg's Liquid Aminos or soy sauce
1½ tablespoons fresh lime juice
1 cup sliced carrots
1 cup chopped snow peas
1 cup chopped zucchini
½ cup chopped jarred roasted red bell peppers, drained
½ cup black beans, rinsed and drained
½ cup canned chickpeas, rinsed and drained
2 cups cooked wild rice
  Avocado slices
  Chopped macadamia nuts

Recipe Notes
- Use cooked brown rice instead of wild rice.
- Sprinkle each serving with unsweetened coconut flakes before serving.
- Experiment with a variety of vegetable combinations, such as asparagus, broccoli, green bell peppers, and/or sweet peas.

Heat olive oil in large skillet over medium heat. Stir in onions, and cook until soft and translucent. Add garlic, and cook for 30 seconds, stirring constantly so garlic doesn't burn. Add ½ cup pineapple juice, Bragg's Liquid Aminos, and lime juice. Stir in carrots, snow peas, zucchini, red peppers, black beans, and chickpeas. Increase heat to medium high, stirring often. Cook 5 minutes, or until ¾ of the liquid is absorbed and vegetables are slightly softened. Add wild rice and pineapple. Increase heat, and stir-fry until heated through. Serve immediately. Garnish with avocado slices and chopped macadamia nuts.

> Bragg's Liquid Aminos is an alternative to soy sauce that has no added salt or preservatives. Bragg's Liquid Aminos is a certified non-GMO (not genetically modified) liquid protein concentrate, derived from healthy soybeans, that contains sixteen essential and nonessential amino acids.

Chipotle Black Bean Burgers

1 (15-ounce) can black beans, rinsed and drained
1 cup mashed cooked sweet potatoes (about 1 large sweet potato, peeled)
¼ cup oat flour (see Recipe Notes)
½ tablespoon dried parsley
¼ teaspoon chipotle chili pepper seasoning
¼ teaspoon garlic powder
¼ teaspoon salt
⅛ teaspoon pepper

YIELD: 6 servings
SERVING SIZE: 1 burger

Preheat oven to broil setting. With a potato masher or fork, mash black beans in a large bowl, leaving about ¼ of the beans whole. Mix in sweet potatoes, oat flour, parsley, chipotle chili pepper seasoning, garlic powder, salt, and pepper. Scoop out ⅓ cup of bean mixture, and place on an 11 by 17-inch baking sheet that has been rubbed with olive oil. Flatten and shape into a circle with spatula. Repeat with the remaining bean mixture to make 6 burgers.

Broil 4 inches from heat about 7 – 8 minutes or until golden brown. Flip burgers carefully with spatula. Broil 2 – 3 more minutes, and serve.

Recipe Notes
• Spread burger with Guacamole with a Little Kick.
• Top with tomato slices, lettuce, and/or onions.
• Make your own oat flour by placing old-fashioned rolled oats in a food processor or blender and process until fine (1 cup old-fashioned oats will yield about ¾ cup ground oats).

Chipotle (pronounced "chee-POAT-lay") is a smoke-dried jalapeno chili used primarily in Mexican and Mexican-inspired cuisine, such as Mexican-American and Tex-Mex. Chipotle chili pepper is considered to be medium in heat compared with other chilies.

Main Dishes

Coconut Rice

YIELD: 8 servings
SERVING SIZE:
   about 1 cup

1 cup brown rice

1 cup wild rice

2 cups water

1 (14-ounce) can unsweetened coconut milk (about 2 cups)

3 cups diced, cooked sweet potatoes, peeled (about 2 – 3 potatoes)

1 cup sweet peas, cooked

1 cup canned black beans, rinsed and drained

¼ cup chopped green onions

2 tablespoons fresh lime juice

½ teaspoon ground ginger

¼ teaspoon salt

⅛ teaspoon pepper

Rinse rice in a fine mesh sieve to remove the surface starches. (They're what make rice sticky.) Mix water, coconut milk, and rice in a large saucepan. Heat to boiling. Reduce heat to simmer, stirring occasionally. Cook, uncovered, until liquid evaporates, about 40 – 45 minutes.

While rice is cooking, prepare the rest of the ingredients. Keep vegetables and beans warm. When rice is finished, add ingredients to rice. Stir well, and serve immediately.

Recipe Notes
• Mix in chopped macadamia nuts before serving.
• Substitute carrots or butternut squash for sweet potatoes.

Coconut milk is a thick, milky-white liquid made by extracting the fat from grated coconut meat. It should not be confused with coconut water, which is the liquid that comes out of a cracked coconut. Considered by some to be a miracle food, coconut milk provides a boost to the body's immune system. It is anticarcinogenic, antimicrobial, antibacterial, and antiviral. Coconut milk is also a dairy-free alternative for people who are lactose intolerant.

Delicata Squash with Kale and Beans

1 recipe Delicata Squash Rings (p. 141)
1 tablespoon extra-virgin olive oil
1 cup chopped onion
1 clove garlic, minced
½ cup water or Vegetable Broth (p. 134)
1 (15-ounce) can cannellini beans, rinsed and drained
4 cups chopped kale, stems removed
½ teaspoon dried thyme
1 tablespoon chopped fresh parsley or 1 teaspoon dried parsley

YIELD: **6 servings**
SERVING SIZE:
about 1 cup

Prepare Delicata Squash Rings according to directions. During the last 10 minutes of cooking time, heat olive oil in large skillet over medium heat. Add onions, and cook about 5 minutes or until soft and translucent. Stir in garlic, and cook 30 seconds, stirring constantly so garlic doesn't burn. Pour in water or broth, beans, kale, thyme, and parsley. Stir well, and cover. Cook 3 – 5 minutes or until kale is slightly wilted.

Remove squash rings from oven. Cut into 1-inch cubes, and add to skillet. Cook 5 more minutes, and serve.

Recipe Notes
• Substitute great northern beans for cannellini beans.
• Use fresh spinach instead of kale.
• Add 1½ – 2 cups cooked brown rice or wild rice.

> Any winter squash works well in this recipe, but I must say that delicata squash is my favorite. Delicata squash is an oblong winter squash with cream-colored, green-striped skin and a golden inner flesh.

Main Dishes

Flatbread Pizza with Macadamia Nut Cheese

YIELD: 8 servings
SERVING SIZE: 1 slice

Pizza

2½   cups whole wheat flour

2   tablespoons flaxseed meal

1   teaspoon salt

1   cup warm water

1   cup Spinach-Artichoke Dip (p. 97)

1   cup Classic Tomato Sauce (p. 140)

Macadamia Nut Cheese

½   cup raw macadamia nuts

Toppings

Green peppers, mushrooms, black olives, onions, roasted red bell peppers

Mix flour, flaxseed meal, salt, and water in a food processor until dough forms a ball. Turn dough onto a floured work surface, and knead for 5 minutes. Transfer to a bowl, and cover tightly with plastic wrap. Let dough rest at room temperature for 30 minutes.

Preheat oven to 450 degrees. Rub a little flour on a rolling pin, and roll dough out onto a preheated pizza stone or an oiled pizza pan into a 12-inch or 14-inch circle (depending on the thickness of crust you prefer). If dough is too sticky to roll, put some flour on your fingertips and press dough to edges. With a fork, poke holes all across crust dough. Bake 10 minutes, and remove from oven.

Recipe Notes
- Substitute Pesto for Spinach-Artichoke Dip.

Spread Spinach Artichoke Dip across crust, and top with Classic Tomato Sauce. Add desired toppings. Bake 20 minutes or until edges of crust are brown and slightly crispy. Remove from oven, and let sit 5 minutes before slicing and serving. While pizza is cooling, place ½ cup of macadamia nuts in a food processor until finely ground like grated Parmesan cheese. Sprinkle on top of cooked pizza, and serve.

> Macadamia nuts are highly nutritious with a smooth, rich, buttery taste. They also have the highest amount of beneficial monounsaturated fats of any nut.

Garden Quinoa

½ cup quinoa
1 cup water
½ tablespoon extra-virgin olive oil
½ cup diced red onion
1–2 cloves garlic, minced (use 2 for a strong garlic flavor)
½ cup chopped asparagus spears
½ cup diced red bell peppers
½ cup diced tomatoes, unpeeled, unseeded
2 tablespoons pine nuts
¼ cup chopped fresh parsley
1½ tablespoons chopped fresh oregano or 1 teaspoon dried oregano flakes
¼ teaspoon salt

YIELD: 6 servings
SERVING SIZE:
about ½ cup

Rinse quinoa under cold running water in a fine mesh sieve until water runs clear. Transfer quinoa to a small saucepan, and add water. Heat to boiling. Reduce heat to low, and cover. Simmer gently with lid tilted for 20 minutes or until nearly all of the liquid is absorbed.

While quinoa is cooking, heat olive oil in a large skillet over medium heat. Add onion and cook until soft and translucent. Stir in garlic, and cook for 30 seconds, stirring constantly so garlic doesn't burn. Add asparagus, red peppers, and tomatoes, squeezing tomatoes with your hands to release their juices into the skillet. Cook over low heat for 5–8 minutes.

Add cooked quinoa to skillet, and stir in pine nuts, parsley, oregano, and salt. Stir well, and cook until heated thoroughly and serve.

> While quinoa is usually considered to be a whole grain, it's actually a seed. However, it can be prepared and used like a whole grain, such as brown rice.

Recipe Notes
- Can also be served as a cold side dish or as a topping for a lettuce salad.
- Stir in ¼ cup Avocado-Tomato Salad Dressing, Italian Salad Dressing, or Lemon-Tahini Salad Dressing.
- Other vegetable ideas are artichokes, broccoli, carrots, celery, green beans, and/or mushrooms.

Main Dishes

Greek-Style Stuffed Peppers

YIELD: 6 servings
SERVING SIZE:
about 2 pepper
halves

1 tablespoon extra-virgin olive oil
½ cup chopped onion
½ cup diced zucchini
1 clove garlic, minced
1 (8-ounce) can tomato sauce
3 chopped canned artichokes, drained
½ cup chopped black olives
1 teaspoon dried oregano flakes or 1 tablespoon chopped fresh oregano
1 teaspoon dried parsley or 1 tablespoon chopped fresh parsley
½ teaspoon salt
6 medium bell peppers (green, orange, red, and/or yellow)
2 cups cooked quinoa
1½ tablespoons pine nuts

Preheat oven to 350 degrees. Place artichokes in a food processor, and pulse until artichokes are chopped well. Set aside. Heat olive oil over medium heat. Add onion and zucchini. Cook 3 – 5 minutes or until vegetables are softened. Lower heat, and add garlic. Cook 30 seconds, stirring constantly so garlic doesn't burn. Add tomato sauce, artichokes, olives, oregano, parsley, and salt. Cook 15 minutes, or until sauce is thickened.

While sauce is cooking, prepare peppers. Cut in half lengthwise, and remove stems and seeds. Place peppers in boiling water for 5 minutes. Drain in colander, and place in a large baking dish, cut side up. When sauce is finished, mix in the quinoa and pine nuts. Stir well. Spoon mixture evenly into pepper halves. Add hot water to dish to a depth of ½ inch. Bake uncovered for 20 minutes.

Recipe Notes
• Increase the protein content of this dish by adding 1 (15-ounce) can great northern beans or pinto beans, rinsed and drained.
• Use brown rice or couscous instead of quinoa.
• Add chopped fresh spinach leaves.

> Bell peppers, also known as sweet peppers, are beautifully shaped, glossy in appearance, and come in a variety of vivid colors such as green, red, yellow, orange, purple, brown, and black. Bite into a fresh bell pepper, and you will find a refreshingly sweet, crunchy texture. Green and purple peppers tend to be the most bitter, while the red, orange, and yellow varieties are sweeter and almost fruity.

Grilled Portabello Steaks
with Sun-Dried Tomato Tofu

YIELD: 4 servings
SERVING SIZE:
  1 mushroom cap and
  2 ounces of tofu

4   portabello mushroom caps

Marinade

¼   cup extra-virgin olive oil

¼   cup unsweetened pineapple juice or orange juice

¼   cup Bragg's Liquid Aminos or soy sauce

2   tablespoons chopped green onions (green parts only)

1   clove garlic, minced

½   teaspoon dried crushed rosemary

Sun-Dried Tomato Tofu

8   ounces extra-firm tofu, cut into ½-inch rectangular slices
    (2 ounces each)

1   tablespoon extra-virgin olive oil

¼   cup chopped sun-dried tomatoes, packed in oil, drained

¼   cup sliced black olives

2   tablespoons chopped fresh basil

2   tablespoons chopped fresh parsley

⅛   teaspoon garlic powder

Place mushrooms in a glass dish with gills up. Whisk together marinade ingredients in a small bowl, and pour over caps. Marinate at room temperature 30 minutes.

While mushrooms marinate, prepare Sun-Dried Tomato Tofu. Place tofu slices in an 8 by 8-inch baking dish, and drizzle with olive oil. Top with sun-dried tomatoes and olives. Add basil, parsley, and garlic powder. Let sit at room temperature 30 minutes. Preheat oven to broil setting while tofu marinates. Put tofu in the oven and broil for 5 – 7 minutes.

Preheat barbecue grill. When grill is ready, place mushroom caps over heat for 5 minutes, flipping halfway through cooking time.

To serve, place grilled mushroom caps on a plate, top with tofu slices, and drizzle a tablespoon or two of the rosemary marinade over all.

Main Dishes

Recipe Notes

- Substitute ¼ cup chopped roasted red bell peppers for the sun-dried tomatoes.
- Use chopped fresh oregano instead of basil.
- Add chopped canned artichokes or diced onions to the tofu slices.
- Bragg's Liquid Aminos is an alternative to soy sauce that has no added salt or preservatives. Bragg's Liquid Aminos is a certified non-GMO (not genetically modified) liquid protein concentrate, derived from healthy soybeans, that contains sixteen essential and nonessential amino acids.

> Portabello (or portobella) mushrooms are easy to identify because of their large size, which is at least four inches in diameter. They are mostly eaten broiled and grilled, but they can also be baked or sautéed. Portabellos are often used as a replacement for hamburgers in vegan or vegetarian recipes.

Hummus Casserole

YIELD: 10 servings
SERVING SIZE: about ½ cup

1 recipe Hummus (p. 92)
½ cup water
1 carrot, shredded (about 1 cup)
1 cup cooked chopped spinach, squeezed dry
1 cup diced zucchini, unpeeled
¼ cup chopped green onions (green parts only)
½ teaspoon salt
2 cups cooked brown rice

Preheat oven to 350 degrees. Prepare Hummus according to directions and place in a large bowl. (You will use the entire recipe.) Add water, carrots, spinach, zucchini, green onions, salt, and brown rice. Stir well. Pour into a 9 by 13-inch casserole dish that has been lightly rubbed with olive oil. Bake, covered, for 20 minutes.

Recipe Notes

- Substitute quinoa or couscous for the brown rice.
- Use Confetti Hummus.

- Omit the baking step, and use as a dip for fresh vegetables.
- Serve with Flatbread or Tortilla Chips.

> Hummus is a thick spread made from chickpeas, olive oil, garlic, and tahini. It can be used as a dip or a sauce.

Lentil-Spinach "Meatballs"

½ cup dry lentils, sorted and rinsed

1½ cups Vegetable Broth (p. 134) or water

½ cup diced onion, divided

1 clove garlic, minced

1½ teaspoons extra-virgin olive oil

1 cup finely chopped white button mushrooms

½ (10-ounce) package frozen chopped spinach, thawed, squeezed dry

½ cup oat flour (see Recipe Notes)

2 tablespoons finely chopped walnuts

2 tablespoons flaxseed meal

1 teaspoon dried basil

1 teaspoon dried parsley

½ teaspoon garlic powder

½ teaspoon salt

YIELD: 8 servings
SERVING SIZE: 2 balls

Place lentils and broth in a medium saucepan and bring to a boil. Lower heat, and add ¼ cup onions, and garlic. Cover, and simmer with lid tilted for 45 minutes. While lentils cook, heat olive oil over medium-low heat in a large skillet. Add ¼ cup onions, mushrooms, and spinach, and stir to coat. Cook 5 minutes, stirring frequently. Set aside.

When lentils are done cooking, drain any water that remains and stir into mixture of onions, mushrooms, and spinach. Add oat flour, walnuts, flaxseed meal, basil, parsley, garlic powder, and salt. Stir well. Transfer to a food processor or blender, and process 10 – 15 seconds or until smooth. Form mixture into balls (about 2 tablespoons per ball), and place on an 11 by 17-inch baking dish that has been rubbed with olive oil. Bake 30 minutes.

Main Dishes

Recipe Notes

- To sort lentils, spread them in a single layer on an 11 by 17-inch baking sheet. Look for discolored and misshapen beans, and discard any unwanted debris. Place good lentils into a colander and rinse thoroughly using cold water.
- Make your own oat flour by placing old-fashioned rolled oats in a food processor or blender and process until fine (1 cup old-fashioned oats will yield about ¾ cup ground oats).
- Serve as an appetizer or as part of a main dish.
- Add brown rice, spaghetti squash, or whole grain pasta and Classic Tomato Sauce to make Daniel Fast spaghetti and meatballs.
- Flatten meatballs and stuff into Whole Grain Tortillas that have been spread with Hummus.

> Flaxseed meal is a powder made from ground flaxseeds. It can be found in health food stores and some grocery stores. Instead of buying flaxseed meal, you can also grind whole flaxseeds at home using a coffee or seed grinder.

Marinated Tofu

YIELD: 4 servings
SERVING SIZE: about 2 ounces

8   ounces extra-firm tofu, drained
¼   cup unsweetened pineapple juice
2   tablespoons Bragg's Liquid Aminos or soy sauce
1   clove garlic, minced

Slice tofu into 1-inch cubes and place in an 8 by 8-inch baking dish. Mix pineapple juice, Bragg's Liquid Aminos or soy sauce, and garlic in a small bowl. Use a whisk to combine. Pour over tofu, and put in refrigerator to marinate 30 – 45 minutes.

Preheat oven to 350 degrees. Bake (in same dish) for 20 minutes or until the outside is a deep, golden brown and slightly crispy.

Recipe Notes

- Use to make Sesame Vegetables with Rice and Tofu.
- Bragg's Liquid Aminos is an alternative to soy sauce that has no added salt or preservatives. Bragg's Liquid Aminos is a certified non-GMO (not genetically modified) liquid protein concentrate,

derived from healthy soybeans, that contains sixteen essential and nonessential amino acids.

> Tofu, or bean curd, is a soft white food made by coagulating soy milk and then pressing the resulting curds into blocks. Because of its cheeselike texture, tofu is often substituted for meats, cheeses, and certain dairy products.

Mexican Rice and Beans

1½ cups brown rice
1 tablespoon extra-virgin olive oil
1 cup diced red onion
2 cloves garlic, minced
2½ cups water
1 (10-ounce) can diced tomatoes and green chilies, undrained
1 teaspoon cumin
¼ teaspoon cayenne pepper
1 (15-ounce) can black beans, rinsed and drained
1 tablespoon chopped fresh parsley or 1 teaspoon dried parsley

YIELD: 6 servings
SERVING SIZE:
about 1 cup

Rinse rice in a fine mesh sieve under cold running water for 30 seconds, swirling the rice around with your hand. Drain, and set aside. Heat olive oil in a large saucepan over medium heat. Add onions and cook until soft and translucent. Add garlic, and cook 30 seconds, stirring constantly so garlic doesn't burn.

Pour in water, rice, tomatoes, chilies, cumin, and cayenne pepper. Heat to boiling. Reduce heat and cover. Simmer 45 – 55 minutes or until rice is tender and nearly all of the liquid is absorbed. Add beans, and stir well. Cook another 8 – 10 minutes. Add parsley, and serve.

Recipe Notes
• This recipe is fairly spicy; to cut down on the heat, reduce cayenne pepper to ⅛ teaspoon or eliminate it completely.
• Spread on Broiled Polenta Squares, and top with avocado slices.

> Brown rice is a complex carbohydrate, making it a good source of energy. Beans provide protein, fiber, and iron. Putting the two together in one dish results in a well-balanced meal and a complete protein, which means all of the nine essential amino acids are included.

Main Dishes

Purple Sticky Rice with Cashews

YIELD: 6 servings

SERVING SIZE:
about 1 cup

2 cups Thai black rice

1 (14-ounce) can unsweetened coconut milk (about 2 cups)

½ cup water

½ teaspoon salt

1 tablespoon extra-virgin olive oil

1 cup thinly sliced red onion, sliced pole to pole (see Recipe Notes)

1 cup cooked sweet peas

½ cup cashew halves and pieces, toasted

1 tablespoon sesame seeds

Rinse rice in a fine mesh sieve, and place in a large saucepan. Add coconut milk, water, and salt. Stir to combine. Cook over medium-high heat to bring to a boil. Reduce heat to low, and cover. Cook 20 minutes. Stir well. Cover again, and cook an additional 15 – 20 minutes. Nearly all of the liquid should be absorbed.

While rice is cooking, heat olive oil in a small skillet over medium to medium-low heat. Add onions and stir to coat. Cook 20 minutes or until onions are slightly browned and crispy, stirring frequently.

Add cooked peas and cashews to rice, and stir. Place a mound of rice on each serving plate, and sprinkle with sesame seeds. Top with onions.

Recipe Notes
- Add 1 cup canned chickpeas, drained, to boost the protein content.
- Substitute 1 cup cut green beans or chopped broccoli for peas.
- To slice an onion pole to pole, or into half rings, think of the onion as a globe. Trim root end (south pole) and stem end (north pole). Peel off outer layers. Cut onion in half from north pole to south pole, making a series of vertical slices perpendicular to the equator of the onion.
- Another way to cook this recipe is to steam or boil the rice in water. Add cooked rice, along with coconut milk and peas, to onions once they have become slightly browned. Mix well, and cook 15 minutes, or until nearly most of the coconut milk has been absorbed, stirring frequently.
- Most health food stores and some large supermarket chains carry both Thai black rice and coconut milk.

Thai black rice, or purple sticky rice, has a sweet flavor, sticky texture, and deep purple color when cooked. It is commonly used as a dessert rice in Southeast Asia.

Rice and Cabbage Casserole

½ tablespoon extra-virgin olive oil

½ cup chopped onion

2 cloves garlic, minced

1 cup chopped white button mushrooms

1 (15-ounce) can black beans, rinsed and drained

2 (14.5-ounce) cans diced tomatoes, undrained

2 tablespoons chopped fresh parsley

1 teaspoon dried oregano flakes

1 teaspoon salt

⅛ teaspoon pepper

4 cups chopped green cabbage

1 cup cooked brown or wild rice

YIELD: 8 servings
SERVING SIZE:
   about 1 cup

Mash 1 cup black beans, and set aside. Heat olive oil over medium heat in a large skillet. Add onions, and cook until soft and translucent. Stir in garlic, mushrooms, mashed beans, tomatoes, parsley, oregano, salt, and pepper. Reduce heat to low, and cook 20 minutes, stirring occasionally.

Preheat oven to 350 degrees. Steam cabbage 8 – 10 minutes or until crisp tender (or add cabbage to boiling water, and cook 5 – 7 minutes). Lightly rub a 9 by 13-inch baking dish with olive oil, and cover bottom of dish with cooked cabbage. Place remaining whole beans and rice on top of cabbage. Pour tomato mixture over all. Bake 20 minutes.

Recipe Notes
- Add 1 cup diced zucchini.
- Substitute cooked quinoa for the brown rice.
- Use 1 (14.5-ounce can) tomato puree and ¼ cup water in place of the diced tomatoes.

Main Dishes

Cabbage has a round shape and is composed of superimposed leaf layers. It is in the same vegetable family as Brussels sprouts, broccoli, and kale. There are three major types of cabbage: green, red, and savoy. Two other cabbage varieties are bok choy and Chinese (or napa) cabbage.

Romaine Wraps

YIELD: 2 servings
SERVING SIZE:
about 2 stuffed
leaves

4   romaine lettuce hearts or leaves

½   cup Hummus (p. 92)

¼   cup cucumber slices, cut ¼-inch thick and into half-moons

¼   cup shredded carrots

¼   cup chopped zucchini

½   yellow bell pepper, julienned

Spread 2 tablespoons of hummus on each leaf. Top with cucumber, carrots, zucchini, and pepper. Eat like a taco, or roll up like a tortilla (depending on the size and shape of the leaf).

Recipe Notes
• Substitute bok choy leaves for the romaine leaves.
• Use Confetti Hummus.
• Other topping ideas are artichokes, avocado, beans, cooked brown rice, broccoli, green peppers, mushrooms, olives, onions, red peppers, sunflower seeds, and/or tomatoes.

> Romaine lettuce usually works the best for wraps because their large, sturdy leaves hold ingredients well.

Sesame Vegetables with Rice and Tofu

YIELD: 4 servings
SERVING SIZE:
about 1¼ cups

1   tablespoon extra-virgin olive oil

1   cup chopped onion

1   clove garlic, minced

¼   cup unsweetened pineapple juice or water

⅛   cup Bragg's Liquid Aminos or soy sauce

½   tablespoon tahini

½ teaspoon ground ginger

1½ cups cooked wild rice

1 recipe Marinated Tofu (p. 172)

2 cups chopped steamed broccoli florets

1 cup chopped steamed carrots

¼ cup toasted chopped walnuts

2 teaspoons sesame seeds

Prepare Marinated Tofu as directed and set aside. Heat olive oil in a large skillet over medium heat, and add onions. Cook until onions are soft and translucent. Stir in garlic, and cook 30 seconds, stirring constantly so garlic doesn't burn. Mix pineapple juice, Bragg's Liquid Aminos, tahini, and ginger in a small bowl. Use a whisk to combine, and pour into skillet. Add rice, tofu, broccoli, and carrots, and cook, covered, about 5 minutes or until heated through. Sprinkle with walnuts and sesame seeds. Stir, and serve.

Recipe Notes

- Add 1 cup canned chickpeas, drained.
- Stir in about ½ teaspoon finely diced fresh ginger root for extra flavor.
- Other vegetable ideas are chopped red bell peppers, snow peas, or zucchini.
- Bragg's Liquid Aminos is an alternative to soy sauce that has no added salt or preservatives. Bragg's Liquid Aminos is a certified non-GMO (not genetically modified) liquid protein concentrate, derived from healthy soybeans, that contains sixteen essential and nonessential amino acids.

Sesame seeds are tiny, flat oval seeds that add a nutty taste and delicate crunch to this recipe.

South of the Border Pizza

YIELD: 4 servings
SERVING SIZE:
about 2 slices

Crust

1½ cups cornmeal

1 cup whole wheat flour

1 cup warm water

1 tablespoon extra-virgin olive oil

½ teaspoon cumin

⅛ teaspoon cayenne pepper

Sauce

1 (15-ounce) can pinto beans, undrained

2 cloves garlic, minced

½ teaspoon onion powder

Toppings

1 cup Salsa (p. 96), drained

1 (14.5-ounce) can corn kernels, drained and roasted (see Recipe Notes)

4 ounces Taco Tofu Crumbles (optional)

½ cup chopped jarred roasted red bell peppers

½ cup sliced black olives

¼ cup diced onion

¼ teaspoon cumin

Taco Tofu Crumbles

8 ounces extra-firm tofu, cut into small cubes

½ tablespoon extra-virgin olive oil

½ teaspoon cumin

½ teaspoon garlic powder

¼ teaspoon salt

⅛ teaspoon cayenne pepper

Preheat oven to 450 degrees. Mix crust ingredients together in a large bowl or food processor until dough forms a ball. Rub a little flour on a rolling pin, and roll dough into a 12-inch circle on a preheated pizza stone or an oiled pizza pan. If dough is too sticky to roll, put some flour on your fingertips and press dough to edges. With a fork, poke holes all across crust dough. Bake 10 minutes, and remove from oven.

While crust is baking, prepare Taco Tofu Crumbles, if desired. Put cumin, garlic powder, salt, and cayenne pepper in a small bowl, and mix well. Heat olive oil in a skillet, and add tofu. Mix in cumin, garlic power, salt, and cayenne pepper. Cook 2–3 minutes, stirring constantly.

When crust is done, remove from oven and spread pinto bean sauce and salsa on top. Add ½ cup of roasted corn kernels, Taco Tofu Crumbles (optional), roasted red peppers, olives, and onions. Sprinkle cumin over pizza. Bake 15–20 minutes or until edges of crust are brown and slightly crispy. Remove from oven, and let sit 5 minutes before slicing and serving.

Recipe Notes
- To roast corn kernels, place on a lightly oiled 11 by 17-inch baking sheet, and spread out in one layer. Bake at 450 degrees for 10 minutes. Stir well, and return to oven for another 5–10 minutes. Corn should be slightly browned.
- Use the remaining roasted corn kernels in a stir-fry or as a salad topping.
- Add ½ cup canned black beans, drained.
- To make a gluten-free crust, use brown rice flour for the wheat flour, or use all cornmeal.
- For the Taco Tofu Crumbles, add 1 teaspoon Taco Seasoning instead of the suggested spices.

Don't let the ingredients list for South of the Border Pizza intimidate you. Although this is a fairly involved recipe, you can simplify it by doing some of the prep work ahead of time. Mix the pizza dough and let it sit. Cut up the vegetables, and put them in containers. Make the bean sauce and Taco Tofu Crumbles. Now you have half the work already done. All that's left is to assemble the pizza and bake.

Main Dishes

Spaghetti Squash Stir-Fry

YIELD: 4 servings
SERVING SIZE:
about 1 cup

1 tablespoon extra-virgin olive oil

1 cup chopped onion

1 clove garlic, minced

2 cups cooked broccoli, cut into 1-inch florets

2 cups cooked spaghetti squash, cut into 2-inch pieces

1½ cups cooked brown or wild rice

½ cup canned black beans, rinsed and drained

¼ cup Bragg's Liquid Aminos or soy sauce

1 teaspoon dried basil

½ tablespoon tahini

2 tablespoons chopped walnuts or cashews

Heat olive oil in large skillet over medium heat. Add onions, and cook until soft and translucent. Stir in garlic, broccoli, spaghetti squash, rice, beans, Bragg's Liquid Aminos, basil, and tahini. Cook 5 minutes, stirring frequently. Mix in walnuts just before serving.

Recipe Notes
• Substitute chopped zucchini for the broccoli.
• Use cashews instead of walnuts.
• Add ½ cup chopped avocado to the stir-fry.
• Other vegetable ideas are green beans, mushrooms, and/or sweet peas.
• Bragg's Liquid Aminos is an alternative to soy sauce that has no added salt or preservatives. Bragg's Liquid Aminos is a certified non-GMO (not genetically modified) liquid protein concentrate, derived from healthy soybeans, that contains sixteen essential and nonessential amino acids.
• Tahini is a thick paste made from ground sesame seeds. It is a staple in Middle Eastern cooking and can be found at health food stores and most large grocery chains.

To bake a spaghetti squash, preheat oven to 375 degrees. With a fork, prick squash all over and place directly on rack in middle of oven. Cook 1 hour. Remove from oven, and let squash cool 10–15 minutes before cutting in half and removing seeds. Pull a fork lengthwise through the flesh to separate into long strands.

Spinach-Artichoke Pasta with Vegetables

1 pound whole grain pasta
1 tablespoon extra-virgin olive oil
½ cup diced red onion
1 cup chopped canned artichokes, drained, reserve 2 tablepoons juice
1 cup chopped jarred roasted red bell peppers, drained
½ cup chopped black olives
1 recipe Spinach-Artichoke Dip (p. 97)

YIELD: 12 servings
SERVING SIZE:
about 1 cup

Cook pasta according to package directions. While pasta is cooking, heat olive oil over medium heat and add red onions. Cook 3 – 5 minutes, or until onions are soft and translucent. Stir in artichokes, artichoke juice, peppers, and olives. Lower heat and cook until pasta is done.

When pasta is finished cooking, drain. Add Spinach-Artichoke Dip and vegetable mixture to pasta. If desired, add ¼ cup hot water or 1 – 2 tablespoons olive oil to thin sauce before serving. Stir well, and serve.

Recipe Notes
- Substitute 2 cups cooked brown rice for the pasta.
- Other vegetable ideas are chopped broccoli, green beans, mushrooms, and/or tomatoes.

Olives are high in oleic acid, a monounsaturated fat that has been shown to lower blood cholesterol levels. They also provide the body with iron, vitamin E, copper, and dietary fiber.

Spinach-Zucchini Casserole

1 (28-ounce) can diced tomatoes, undrained
2 cloves garlic, minced
½ tablespoon dried basil
½ tablespoon dried oregano flakes
½ tablespoon dried parsley
1 teaspoon salt
1½ pounds zucchini, sliced into ½-inch rounds (about 2 – 3 medium zucchini)
3 cups packed fresh spinach, stems removed
1 cup thinly sliced onion, sliced pole to pole (see Recipe Notes)
  Cooked brown rice, lentils, or quinoa

YIELD: 6 servings
SERVING SIZE:
about 1 cup

Main Dishes

Preheat oven to 350 degrees. Pour tomatoes into small saucepan, and add garlic, basil, oregano, parsley, and salt. Heat to boiling. Reduce heat, and simmer about 10 minutes.

While sauce is cooking, prepare vegetables. Lightly coat a 9 by 13-inch casserole dish with olive oil. Place zucchini rounds on bottom of dish, stacking extra rounds to make a second layer, if needed. Spread spinach leaves and onion slices on top of zucchini. When sauce is done, pour sauce over all, making sure vegetables are coated with tomatoes and their juice. Bake 25 – 30 minutes, or until zucchini is tender. Stir well, and serve with cooked brown rice, lentils, or quinoa.

Recipe Notes
- Serve alone or as a side dish.
- Add ½ cup shredded carrots, chopped mushrooms, chopped black olives, or chopped yellow squash.
- To slice an onion pole to pole, think of the onion as a globe. Trim root end (south pole) and stem end (north pole). Peel off outer layers. Cut onion in half from north pole to south pole, making a series of vertical slices perpendicular to the equator of the onion.

> When choosing zucchini, look for ones that are firm and slender with a bright green color. Avoid zucchini that has wrinkled skin and soft spots. Store zucchini in the crisper drawer of the refrigerator, and wash just before using.

Stuffed Acorn Squash

YIELD: 4 servings
SERVING SIZE: ½ acorn squash with filling

2 acorn squash, unpeeled
½ cup quinoa
1½ cups unsweetened apple juice or water
1 cup chopped apples, unpeeled
1 teaspoon ground cinnamon

¼ teaspoon ground cloves

¼ teaspoon ground nutmeg

¼ cup chopped pecans

¼ cup raisins

¼ cup golden raisins

Preheat oven to 375 degrees. Cut squash in half lengthwise, and scoop out seeds. Place halves, cut side down, in a large baking dish. Pour in water until it's about ¼-inch deep. Bake 40 minutes.

While squash is cooking, rinse quinoa under cold running water in a fine mesh sieve until water runs clear. Transfer quinoa to a small saucepan, and add apple juice or water, cinnamon, ground cloves, and nutmeg. Heat to boiling. Reduce heat to low, and cover. Simmer gently with lid tilted for 20 minutes or until nearly all of the liquid is absorbed. Stir in pecans and raisins, and set aside until squash is done.

Remove squash from oven, and turn halves over. Stuff each squash half with about ½ cup apple-quinoa mixture. (Depending on the size of the squash, you may have some mixture left over, which makes a great side dish.) Bake 10 minutes.

Recipe Notes
• Substitute brown rice for the quinoa.
• Use ¼ cup chopped dates and ¼ cup chopped dried apricots instead of the raisins.
• Sprinkle each stuffed squash half with unsweetened shredded coconut just before serving.
• Enjoy as a warm breakfast or dessert.

Acorn squash is a small winter squash shaped like an acorn. The most popular variety has dark green skin with distinct ribs and is speckled with orange patches. Inside the acorn squash is a yellow-orange flesh that tastes sweet, nutty, and slightly peppery.

Main Dishes

Tahini Wild Rice Cakes

1½ cups cooked wild rice

2 tablespoons oat flour (see Recipe Notes)

2 tablespoons chopped onion or green onions

1 tablespoon extra-virgin olive oil

1 tablespoon tahini

1 tablespoon chopped fresh parsley or 1 teaspoon dried parsley

¼ teaspoon salt

Avocado slices

Combine all ingredients, except avocado slices, in a large bowl, and stir well. Heat olive oil in large skillet over medium-high heat. Scoop out ⅓ cup of mixture for each cake, and flatten in the skillet with a spatula. Cook 5 minutes, flip rice cake, and cook another 2 minutes on the other side. Serve warm. Top with avocado, if desired.

Recipe Notes

- Make your own oat flour by placing old-fashioned rolled oats in a food processor or blender and process until fine (1 cup old-fashioned oats will yield about ¾ cup ground oats).
- Tahini is a thick paste made from ground sesame seeds. It is a staple in Middle Eastern cooking and can be found at health food stores and most large grocery chains.
- Rice cakes will pack and hold together better if the rice is warm.
- Top with Salsa or Guacamole with a Little Kick.
- Substitute brown rice for wild rice or use a combination of both.
- Serve as a side dish with soup or salad.

> Tahini is a thick paste made from ground sesame seeds. It is a staple in Middle Eastern cooking and can be found at health food stores and most large grocery chains.

Two-Bean Burger

- 1 teaspoon extra-virgin olive oil
- 2 tablespoons chopped onion
- 1 cup canned black beans, rinsed and drained
- 1 cup canned great northern beans, rinsed and drained
- 2 tablespoons flaxseed meal
- 1 teaspoon garlic powder
- ¼ teaspoon cumin
- ¼ teaspoon salt

YIELD: 4 servings
SERVING SIZE: 1 burger

Mash beans in a large bowl, leaving about ¼ of the beans whole, and set aside.

Heat olive oil in large skillet over medium heat. Add onions, and cook until soft and translucent. Place in a bowl with beans, and add flaxseed meal, garlic powder, cumin, and salt.

Return skillet to medium heat, and add a teaspoon of olive oil, if needed, to prevent burgers from sticking. Scoop out about ⅓ cup of bean mixture for each burger, and add to skillet. Flatten with a spatula. Cook 5 minutes, or until bottoms are browned and slightly crispy. Flip, and cook another 5 minutes.

Recipe Notes

- Stir in ¼ cup cooked brown rice for more texture.
- Spread burger with Guacamole with a Little Kick.
- Top with tomato slices, lettuce, and/or onions.
- Try with Taco Seasoning or chili seasoning instead of using cumin, garlic powder, and salt.
- Substitute 2 tablespoons oat flour for the flaxseed meal. Make your own oat flour by placing old-fashioned rolled oats in a food processor or blender and process until fine (½ cup old-fashioned oats will yield about ½ cup ground oats).

The mix of black beans and great northern beans gives this burger a thick, meaty taste.

Main Dishes

Whole Grain Tortillas

YIELD: 8 servings
SERVING SIZE: 1 tortilla

2 cups whole wheat flour

½ cup brown rice or soy flour

2 tablespoons flaxseed meal (optional)

1 teaspoon salt

1 cup warm water

Mix flours, flaxseed meal, salt, and water in a food processor until dough forms a ball. Turn dough onto a floured work surface, and knead for 5 minutes. Transfer to a bowl, and cover tightly with plastic wrap. Let dough sit at room temperature 30 minutes.

Divide dough into 8 equal pieces, and roll each piece into an 8-inch circle about ¼-inch thick on a floured surface. Rub a skillet with olive oil, and set over medium-low heat. Cook tortilla for 1 minute. Turn over and cook 2–3 minutes on second side or until tortilla bubbles up. Repeat for remaining tortillas.

Recipe Notes
- Spread tortilla with Confetti Hummus, Great Northern Dip, Hummus, Pesto, or Spinach-Artichoke Dip, and stuff with beans, rice, and/or vegetables.
- Fill with Black Bean Chili Bake or Taco Salad.
- Instead of brown rice flour, use another whole grain flour, such as amaranth, barley, oat, quinoa, or spelt.
- Flaxseed meal is a powder made from ground flaxseeds. It can be found in health food stores and some grocery stores. Instead of buying flaxseed meal, you can also grind whole flaxseeds at home using a coffee or seed grinder.

> Whole grain foods have all three parts of the grain: the bran, the endosperm, and the germ. Whole grains are a good source of B vitamins, vitamin E, magnesium, iron, and fiber, as well as other valuable antioxidants not found in some fruits and vegetables. You can identify whether a product is whole grain by looking at the ingredients list. If the food is high in a whole grain, the grain will be the first ingredient listed. Also, look for the word *whole* in front of a grain. For example "whole wheat flour" is a whole grain, but "wheat flour" is not.

Wild Rice and Almond Casserole

1 tablespoon extra-virgin olive oil

1 cup wild rice

½ cup chopped green onions (green parts only)

¼ cup slivered almonds

2 cloves garlic, minced

½ teaspoon salt

3 cups Vegetable Broth (p. 134) or water

YIELD: 6 servings
SERVING SIZE:
about ½ cup

Preheat oven to 350 degrees. Heat olive oil in large skillet over medium heat. Add rice, onions, almonds, garlic, and salt. Cook 3 – 5 minutes or until the rice begins to turn slightly yellow, stirring frequently. Transfer to a 1½ or 2-quart casserole dish, pour in broth, and cover. Bake 1 hour or until liquid is absorbed.

Recipe Notes
• Add 1 cup drained chickpeas to boost the protein content.

Wild rice is a long, dark brown or black seed of an annual marsh grass. Contrary to popular belief, it is not a true rice or grain at all. Wild rice is chewy, nutty, and full of flavor.

Main Dishes

Juices

Note: The recipes in this section are intended to be used with a juicer to make fresh fruit and vegetable juices. However, you can easily convert the juices into smoothies by using a high-powered blender that has the ability to pulverize skins, seeds, and peels of whole foods. You can also use a regular blender; however, you will need to alter the recipes slightly (such as by removing the peels of certain fruits if your blender is not powerful enough to process them completely).

See page 27 to learn a few of the benefits of juicing.

To prepare recipes, feed ingredients through the juicer. If using a blender, process ingredients until smooth. For an extra-creamy consistency, add almond milk, rice milk, soy milk, tofu, or ice cubes.

Yield for all juice recipes: 2 servings (serving size: 8 ounces)

- Cut fruits and vegetables to proper size before you begin feeding them through the juicer.
- Leafy greens should be wrapped around a fruit or vegetable that is high in water content (such as an orange slice or a tomato wedge) to prevent the greens from clogging up the juicer.
- If you're new to juicing, start with a simple recipe you know you will like, such as fresh orange or grape juice, before branching out to something less sweet (such as pure vegetable juices).
- Fresh juice should be consumed immediately for maximum nutritional benefit. If necessary, you can refrigerate it, but be sure to drink the juice within twenty-four hours.

Juices

Apple-Broccoli Blast

3 apples, unpeeled and cut into slices
1 cup broccoli florets (about ½ crown)
1 cup blueberries

Carrot Juice with Fennel and Celery

3 carrots, unpeeled and tops removed
2 stalks of celery, tops included
1 cup chopped fennel bulb

Creamy Mango Delight

1 large mango, pitted and peeled
2 apples, unpeeled and cut into slices (discard cores)
½ cup fresh pineapple, cut into chunks
1 kiwifruit, unpeeled

Everything Green

2 Granny Smith apples, unpeeled and cut into slices
1 cup packed fresh spinach, leaves intact
½ medium cucumber, unpeeled and cut in quarters lengthwise
1 cup green grapes
¼ cup fresh parsley, packed
½ lime, peeled, at room temperature (for easier juicing)

Hello Sunshine Orange Juice

2 oranges, peeled and divided into segments
2 apples, unpeeled and cut into slices (discard cores)
1 cup red seedless grapes

New York-Style Fennel Juice

2 carrots, unpeeled and tops removed
2 tomatoes, quartered
½ fennel bulb, sliced
¼ cup fresh parsley, packed

Orange, Blueberry, and Spinach Twist

2 oranges, peeled and divided into segments
1 cup fresh blueberries
1 cup fresh spinach leaves, packed

Orange-Carrot Juice

2 oranges, peeled and divided into segments
3 carrots, unpeeled and tops removed

Orient Express

3 carrots, unpeeled and tops removed
2 apples, unpeeled and cut into slices (discard cores)
1 (1-inch) slice of ginger root, unpeeled

Rainbow Juice

2 pears, unpeeled and cut into slices (discard cores)
2 oranges, peeled and divided into segments
2 kiwifruit, unpeeled
1 cup strawberries
1 cup red and green seedless grapes

Juices

Refreshing Romaine Salad in a Glass

- 1 cup torn romaine lettuce, packed
- ½ cup broccoli florets (about ½ crown)
- 2 apples, unpeeled and cut into slices (discard cores)
- 1 orange, peeled and divided into segments

Ruby Red Beet Juice

- 1 beet, ends removed and quartered
- 2 oranges, peeled and divided into segments
- 2 apples, unpeeled and cut into slices (discard cores)

Sweet Licorice Juice

- 3 apples, unpeeled and cut into slices (discard cores)
- ½ fennel bulb, sliced

Tangy Apple Delight

- 2 apples, unpeeled and cut into slices (discard cores)
- 1 grapefruit, peeled and divided into segments
- 1 cup red seedless grapes

Tomato Juice

- 2 large tomatoes, quartered
- 2 carrots, unpeeled and tops removed
- 2 stalks of celery, tops included

the
APPENDIXES

Acknowledgments

My Lord and Savior, Jesus Christ: I give all thanks and praise to you, Lord God! Thank you for your faithfulness in completing this good work. May it bring honor and glory — and people — to you.

My husband, Justin: Thank you for always believing in me. Your unwavering support helped me to press on, even when I encountered obstacles or grew weary along the way. Thank you for giving me time to write whenever I needed it and for taste-testing all of my recipes! I can't imagine sharing my life and the fulfillment of this dream without you. I love you so much.

My daughters, Isabelle and Jocelyn: You are both treasures from the Lord. I pray that you always know that nothing is too difficult for God. Mommy's book is evidence of that truth. I love you!

My family and friends: Thank you for continually praying for me over the years as I worked on this project. You have played an important role in the writing of this book through the way you have touched my life. I thank God for you.

My editor, Sandra Vander Zicht: I'm still amazed at how God brought us together. Thank you for catching the vision for this book's potential and for helping me to develop my skills as a writer. Your wealth of knowledge shaped my incomplete thoughts about the Daniel Fast into a powerful source of information.

My other editor, Brian Phipps: Thank you for the many hours you spent fine-tuning my manuscript to make it ready for publication. God has gifted you with an eye for detail and a passion for the written word, and I'm thankful he used your strengths to make this book exactly what he wants it to be.

My marketing director, Tom Dean: Thank you for your wisdom and creative ideas on how to maximize the promotion of this book so that people everywhere can benefit from its message. Thank you, too, for your patience with me as an enthusiastic new author getting her feet wet in the publishing industry!

The editing, marketing, and design teams at Zondervan: Thank you for your commitment to this book and for using your talents to serve the Lord. Even though I may never know your names, I appreciate all the work you have done.

My agent, Les Stobbe: Thank you, Les, for stepping out in faith and trusting that God had something big in mind for this book. When we met, I had no idea how the Lord would use that first critique with you to set his plans in motion. In God's infinite wisdom, he knew exactly who would be the perfect agent for this book. I'm glad he chose you.

Those who contributed Daniel Fast testimonies: Thank you for taking the time to write down what God did in your life through the Daniel Fast. I'm confident he will use your testimonies to encourage many others in their journey.

Fasting FAQs

***Q** Why are whole grains and other foods included when Daniel ate only vegetables?*

A This is a great question, and one that I asked myself when learning about the Daniel Fast for the first time. The food guidelines for the Daniel Fast are based on a combination of two Bible passages. In Daniel 1, Daniel eats only vegetables and drinks only water. In Daniel 10, he abstains from choice food, meat, and wine. Most commentaries believe "choice food" refers to bread and sweets.

Because the Bible doesn't provide details on what Daniel ate, there are often variations in the food guidelines for the modern-day Daniel Fast. For example, some people might adopt a more radical eating plan and eliminate everything but fruits and vegetables for three weeks. Others might choose to include a few more foods, such as eggs or fish. However, the guidelines presented in this book are the most widely accepted for this type of fast.

The most important thing is not that you legalistically adhere to Daniel's diet but that you deny yourself foods you commonly eat and enjoy. Your food choices during the fast might be a little different from someone else's, and

that's fine. Some people may need to be stricter than others so that their fast requires genuine sacrifice. If a person regularly eats whole grains, he or she might want to eliminate them for the twenty-one-day period. For others, adhering to the Daniel Fast food guidelines might be challenging enough. Remember, the most important part of the fast is that you seek the Lord in prayer and grow closer to him. He will lead you and give you wisdom regarding how you need to fast. Try not to get so hung up on what you shouldn't eat that you're robbed of the peace God wants you to experience as you seek him.

***Q** Can I use store-bought items instead of making everything?*

A Yes, there are a number of items you can purchase that fall within the guidelines of the Daniel Fast. For example, if you don't have time to make your own tortilla chips, you can buy a brand that is baked and doesn't contain any sugar, preservatives, or added chemicals (for example, Baked Tostitos). Other packaged foods that you can most likely find at your local health food store or supermarket are hummus, guacamole, salsa, and vegetable broth. However, you will need to read the labels carefully to make sure there aren't any restricted ingredients. Sugar is one ingredient that is added to more foods than you realize. The word *sugar* doesn't always appear in the ingredients list, either. Sometimes it is referred to as corn syrup, dextrose, fructose, glucose, high fructose corn syrup, maltodextrin, molasses, rice syrup, and sucrose. If you have any question as to whether a food is allowed, refer to "Foods to Eat" and "Foods to Avoid" on page 63.

Q *What about going out to eat?*

A Yes, it's possible to eat at a restaurant on the Daniel Fast, but you must do your homework. Look at menus online to see what your options are. Call the restaurant if you have questions about a particular dish and how it's prepared. Sometimes I've taken along my homemade dressing and simply ordered a salad.

Q *How can I tell if a product is whole grain?*

A Look at the ingredients on the label. If something is truly a whole grain, it will be listed as such: 100 percent whole grain, whole grain oats, whole rye, whole wheat, and so on. However, if you see only wheat flour or enriched wheat flour listed, you do not have a whole grain product.

Q *Can I have apple cider vinegar?*

A Apple cider vinegar is made from fermented apple cider. During this process, sugar in the apple cider is broken down by bacteria and yeast into alcohol and then into vinegar. Apple cider vinegar contains acetic acid (like other types of vinegar) and some lactic, citric, and malic acids.

This particular type of vinegar is considered to be a time-honored home remedy for a wide range of health problems. Technically, though, it is not allowed on the Daniel Fast because of the fermentation and yeast used in the process of making it. However, many people choose to modify their fasts a bit to include items such as apple cider vinegar. You should do whatever the Lord is leading you to do. Just remember not to get so focused on what you shouldn't eat that you miss the whole purpose of fasting — to draw near to God and worship him.

Q *Why is salt allowed but not sugar?*

A In Daniel 10, the prophet describes his fast by saying, "I ate no choice food; no meat or wine touched my lips" (Dan. 10:3). Though what is meant by "choice food" is not clear, most commentaries conclude he ate no bread or sweets. *The Message* paraphrase sums up Daniel's description of his fast this way: "I ate only plain and simple food."

Salt is included because it is used as a flavor enhancer for the recipes. Sugar is not included because it is addictive and causes a host of problems when consumed, especially in excess. The same could be said for salt. However, sugar is really more of a treat, a choice food, whereas salt does not seem to fall into that category.

The idea is to simplify the diet and to cut out those foods considered to be choice, which would certainly include sugar. Since the Bible does not address certain foods specifically, we can only do our best to determine which foods should not be included in the fast.

Q *What side effects can I expect?*

A Withdrawal symptoms are common, especially toward the beginning of the fast and particularly if caffeine or sugar are staples in your diet. People who make the mistake of jumping into the fast with the attitude of "no meat, no dairy, no sugar, no problem — it's only for twenty-one days" are in for a rude awakening. They don't realize that because their bodies are used to having such products every day, cravings for those foods will be very strong once they are deprived of them. You may experience headaches, difficulty concentrating, hunger pangs, fatigue, sluggishness, and overall weakness. Usually these side effects disappear after a few days. Some people notice slight stomach distress from the rapid increase in fiber consumption, but that too should subside once your body has adjusted.

Verses to Feed On

When your words came, I ate them; they were my joy and my heart's delight;
for I bear your name, O Lord God Almighty.
— Jeremiah 15:16

The following quotations are just a few of the verses that I refer to when I need encouragement or find myself struggling with doubt or fear. Consider them to be weapons in your spiritual arsenal as you fight the good fight of the faith (1 Tim. 6:12). My recommendation is that you do more than read these verses silently. Say each one aloud. Declare the truth, and stand on it! As you listen to yourself speaking God's Word, you will be strengthened, for "faith comes from hearing, and hearing through the word of Christ" (Rom. 10:17 ESV). Focusing on God's promises instead of your feelings will replace any doubt you might be experiencing with complete confidence in the Lord and his goodness.

Let these morsels of truth nourish your spirit and be a source of strength for you throughout your fast, especially if you become weary and need to be refreshed. Review this list often, and memorize the verses that mean the most to you. As you hide these words in your heart, the Lord will bring them to your mind at the times when you need them most.

Be strong and courageous. Do not be terrified; do not be discouraged, for the Lord your God will be with you wherever you go.
— Joshua 1:9

For the eyes of the Lord range throughout the earth to strengthen those whose hearts are fully committed to him.
— 2 Chronicles 16:9

Those who know your name will trust in you, for you, Lord, have never forsaken those who seek you.
— Psalm 9:10

I call on you, O God, for you will answer me; give ear to me and hear my prayer.
— Psalm 17:6

Hear my voice when I call, O Lord; be merciful to me and answer me. My heart says of you, "Seek his face!" Your face, Lord, I will seek.
— Psalm 27:7 - 8

Because your love is better than life, my lips will glorify you. I will praise you as long as I live and in your name I will lift up my hands. My soul will be satisfied as with the richest of foods; with singing lips my mouth will praise you.
— Psalm 63:3 - 5

You are good, and what you do is good; teach me your decrees.
—*Psalm 119:68*

How sweet are your words to my taste, sweeter than honey to my mouth!
—*Psalm 119:103*

The LORD is near to all who call on him, to all who call on him in truth.
—*Psalm 145:18*

I will praise the LORD all my life; I will sing praise to my God as long as I live.
—*Psalm 146:2*

I am the LORD your God, who teaches you what is best for you, who directs you in the way you should go.
—*Isaiah 48:17*

"For I know the plans I have for you," declares the LORD, "plans to prosper you and not to harm you, plans to give you hope and a future. Then you will call upon me and come and pray to me, and I will listen to you. You will seek me and find me when you seek me with all your heart."
—*Jeremiah 29:11–13*

Call to me and I will answer you and tell you great and unsearchable things you do not know.
—*Jeremiah 33:3*

The LORD is good to those whose hope is in him, to the one who seeks him.
—*Lamentations 3:25*

You have been set free from sin and have become slaves to righteousness.
—*Romans 6:18*

Whether you eat or drink or whatever you do, do it all for the glory of God.
—*1 Corinthians 10:31*

Let us not become weary in doing good, for at the proper time we will reap a harvest if we do not give up.
—*Galatians 6:9*

In him and through faith in him we may approach God with freedom and confidence.
—*Ephesians 3:12*

I can do everything through him who gives me strength.
—*Philippians 4:13*

You have been given fullness in Christ.
—*Colossians 2:10*

Be joyful always; pray continually; give thanks in all circumstances, for this is God's will for you in Christ Jesus.
—*1 Thessalonians 5:16–18*

Now faith is being sure of what we hope for and certain of what we do not see.
—*Hebrews 11:1*

Cast all your anxiety on him because he cares for you.
—*1 Peter 5:7*

His divine power has given us everything we need for life and godliness through our knowledge of him who called us by his own glory and goodness.
—*2 Peter 1:3*

How great is the love the Father has lavished on us, that we should be called children of God! And that is what we are!
—*1 John 3:1*

Daniel Fast Menu Planning Tool

This section of the book supplements the suggested meal plans on pages 65–67 and is designed to help you plan your meals more effectively. In the following pages, you will find the ingredients list, yield information, and serving size for each recipe suggested for weeks 1–3. You will appreciate having everything grouped in one area so that you won't have to flip around in the book quite as much to determine what ingredients are needed to make the recipes in the meal plans.

Meal Planning. Before the fast begins, take a look at the suggested meal plans to determine if you want to use all of the recipes listed or if you want to substitute a few of them with other recipes in the book. After you've created a list of recipes you are interested in, you can go to the individual recipe pages for a closer look.

Grocery Shopping. Once you have finalized your menus, refer to the following pages to create your grocery shopping list each week. A helpful hint that will make your shopping experience more productive is to divide your list into categories, such as "canned items," "fruit," "vegetables," "other," and to organize those categories according to their location in the store. The more prepared you are before you leave the house, the less time you will spend getting the items you need for the week.

Ingredients Lists for the Week 1 Suggested Meal Plan (p. 65)

Note: Page numbers next to recipe titles indicate the page on which you can find the complete recipe in part 3, "The Food." Page numbers within ingredients lists are for the page an ingredients list appears on in this appendix. No recipe variations are given in this section. Refer to the recipes in "The Food" for recipe variations.

Breakfast

Baked Oatmeal (p. 71)

YIELD: 6 servings
SERVING SIZE: 2 squares (2 by 2½ inches)

- 1½ cups old-fashioned rolled oats
- 1½ cups unsweetened almond milk
- ½ cup unsweetened applesauce
- ¼ cup chopped dried apricots
- ¼ cup chopped dates or raisins
- ¼ cup chopped pecans or walnuts
- ½ teaspoon cinnamon
- ¼ teaspoon salt

Nutty Fruit Cereal (p. 77)

YIELD: 1 serving
SERVING SIZE: about 1⅓ cups

- 1 banana, peeled and sliced (about 1 cup)
- ⅓ cup fresh blueberries
- 1 tablespoon chopped almonds
- 1 tablespoon chopped walnuts
- 1 teaspoon unsweetened coconut flakes
- ½ cup unsweetened almond or rice milk

Strawberry-Banana Smoothie (p. 79)

YIELD: 2 servings
SERVING SIZE: about 1 cup

- 4 ounces extra-firm tofu
- ¼ cup unsweetened almond milk
- ¼ cup unsweetened apple juice
- 2 tablespoons Date Honey (p. 204)
- 1 cup sliced strawberries
- 1 frozen banana, peeled, sliced (about 1 cup)

Appetizers and Snacks

Broiled Polenta Squares (p. 83)

YIELD: 9 servings
SERVING SIZE: 2 squares (2½ inches)

- 6 cups water
- 1 tablespoon salt
- 2½ cups yellow cornmeal
- 1 teaspoon dried basil or oregano
- ½ teaspoon garlic powder

Cinnamon Roasted Almonds (p. 85)

YIELD: 8 servings
SERVING SIZE: about ¼ cup

- 2 cups whole almonds
- ½ tablespoon extra-virgin olive oil
- ½ teaspoon cinnamon
- ¼ teaspoon salt

Date Honey (p. 87)

YIELD: 12 servings
SERVING SIZE: about 1 tablespoon

1 cup pitted dates (about 6 – 8 Medjool or
  18 – 20 Deglet Noor)
1 cup water
½ teaspoon cinnamon

Hummus (p. 92)

YIELD: 8 servings
SERVING SIZE: about ¼ cup

1 (15-ounce) can chickpeas, rinsed and
  drained
¼ cup tahini
¼ cup water
2 tablespoons extra-virgin olive oil
2 tablespoons fresh lemon juice
2 cloves garlic, minced
¼ cup fresh parsley, packed
½ teaspoon salt
¼ teaspoon ground cumin

Trail Mix (p. 101)

YIELD: 12 servings
SERVING SIZE: about ¼ cup

1 cup whole raw almonds or Cinnamon
  Roasted Almonds (p. 204)
1 cup cashew halves and pieces
1 cup walnut halves and pieces
½ cup golden raisins
½ cup raisins
¼ cup raw sunflower seeds
¼ cup raw pumpkin seeds (pepitas)

Vegetables

Italian-Style Broccoli (p. 147)

YIELD: 6 servings
SERVING SIZE: about 1 cup

2 – 3 broccoli crowns, cut into florets with
  1-inch stems (about 6 cups)
1 tablespoon extra-virgin olive oil
2 cups halved cherry tomatoes
1 cup chopped fennel bulb
½ cup chopped onion
1 clove garlic, minced
2 tablespoons chopped fresh basil or
  1½ teaspoons dried basil
2 tablespoons pine nuts, toasted

Garlic Spring Peas with Leeks (p. 143)

YIELD: 6 servings
SERVING SIZE: about ½ cup

3 cups water
1 pound fresh or frozen spring peas
1 tablespoon extra-virgin olive oil
½ cup chopped leeks (light green and white
  parts only)
2 cloves garlic, minced
½ teaspoon salt
⅛ teaspoon pepper

Tarragon Roasted Asparagus (p. 157)

YIELD: 6 servings
SERVING SIZE: about 6 – 7 thin spears or 3 – 4
thick spears

1 pound asparagus spears, trimmed (36 – 40
  thin spears or 18 – 20 thick spears)
½ tablespoon extra-virgin olive oil
½ teaspoon dried tarragon
½ teaspoon garlic powder
¼ teaspoon salt

Salads, Soups, and Main Dishes

Mega Greek Salad (p. 106)

YIELD: 6 servings
SERVING SIZE: about 1 cup

- 4 cups torn romaine lettuce
- 1 cup chopped canned artichokes, drained
- 1 cup sliced cherry tomatoes
- 1 cup quartered cucumber slices, peeled
- 1 cup sliced black olives
- ½ cup diced green bell pepper
- ½ cup sliced red onion
- ½ cup chopped fresh parsley

Dressing

- ¼ cup extra-virgin olive oil
- ¼ cup fresh lemon juice
- 2 teaspoons dried oregano flakes
- ½ teaspoon salt
- ⅛ teaspoon pepper

Fig, Pear, and Walnut Salad (p. 104)

YIELD: 4 servings
SERVING SIZE: about 1 cup

- 4 cups torn romaine lettuce, loosely packed
- 1 Bosc pear, unpeeled, sliced thin
- ¼ cup diced dried figs
- ¼ cup chopped walnuts
- 2 tablespoons raw sunflower seeds
- 1 recipe Apple-Cinnamon Salad Dressing (p. 207)

Chunky Potato Soup (p. 124)

YIELD: 6 servings
SERVING SIZE: about 1 cup

- 1 tablespoon extra-virgin olive oil
- ½ cup chopped onion
- 1 cup chopped carrots
- 1 cup chopped celery
- 2 cloves garlic, minced
- 4 cups water or Vegetable Broth (p. 207)
- 3 large russet potatoes, peeled, cubed (about 5 cups)
- 1 bay leaf
- 1 teaspoon salt
- ½ teaspoon thyme
- ⅛ teaspoon pepper
- ½ cup unsweetened almond milk
- 2 tablespoons chopped fresh parsley or 1 teaspoon dried parsley

Tuscan Soup (p. 132)

YIELD: 8 servings
SERVING SIZE: about 1¼ cups

- 1 tablespoon extra-virgin olive oil
- 1 cup diced onion
- 1 cup diced carrots
- 2 cloves garlic, minced
- 6 cups water or Vegetable Broth (p. 207)
- 1 cup dry lentils, sorted and rinsed
- 1 (15-ounce) can cannellini beans, rinsed and drained
- 1 (14.5-ounce) can diced tomatoes, undrained
- ½ (10-ounce) package frozen chopped spinach, unthawed
- ½ tablespoon dried crushed rosemary
- 1 bay leaf
- 1 teaspoon salt
- ⅛ teaspoon pepper

Antipasto Pizza Pie (p. 160)

YIELD: 4 – 6 servings
SERVING SIZE: 1 – 2 slices pie

Crust

3 cups cooked brown rice

2 tablespoons extra-virgin olive oil

¼ cup oat flour (see Recipe Notes)

¼ teaspoon garlic powder

¼ teaspoon onion powder

Sauce

1 (8-ounce) can tomato sauce

1 teaspoon dried basil

1 teaspoon dried oregano flakes

1 teaspoon dried parsley

¼ teaspoon garlic powder

Toppings

¼ cup chopped canned artichokes, drained

¼ cup chopped black olives

¼ cup chopped jarred roasted red bell peppers, drained

2 ounces extra-firm tofu, grated (about ½ cup)

1 tablespoon chopped fresh parsley

Black Bean Chili Bake (p. 161)

YIELD: 6 servings

SERVING SIZE: about 1 cup

2 (15-ounce) cans black beans, rinsed and drained

2 (8-ounce) cans tomato sauce

2 cups cooked brown rice

1 (14.5 ounce) can corn kernels, drained

1 cup chopped jarred roasted red bell peppers, drained (see Recipe Notes)

½ cup diced onion

1 tablespoon chili powder

Romaine Wraps (p. 176)

YIELD: 2 servings

SERVING SIZE: about 2 stuffed leaves

4 romaine lettuce hearts or leaves

½ cup Hummus (p. 205)

¼ cup cucumber slices, cut ¼-inch thick and into half-moons

¼ cup shredded carrots

¼ cup chopped zucchini

½ yellow bell pepper, julienned

Other

Apple-Cinnamon Salad Dressing (p. 113)

YIELD: 8 servings

SERVING SIZE: about 1 tablespoon

¼ cup extra-virgin olive oil

¼ cup unsweetened apple juice

1 tablespoon fresh lemon juice

1 tablespoon diced red onion

¼ teaspoon cinnamon

Vegetable Broth (p. 134)

YIELD: 8 servings

SERVING SIZE: about 1 cup

8 cups water

1 onion, quartered

2 carrots, unpeeled and cut into 2-inch chunks

2 celery stalks, cut into 2-inch chunks, leafy tops included

1 russet potato, unpeeled and cut into 2-inch chunks

4 white button mushrooms, sliced

⅛ cup fresh parsley or ½ tablespoon dried parsley

2 cloves garlic, peeled

1 bay leaf

1 teaspoon dried thyme

1 teaspoon salt

6 peppercorns

Ingredients Lists for the Week 2 Suggested Meal Plan (p. 66)

Note: Page numbers next to recipe titles indicate the page on which you can find the complete recipe in part 3, "The Food." Page numbers within ingredients lists are for the page an ingredients list appears on in this appendix. No recipe variations are given in this section. Refer to the recipes in "The Food" for recipe variations.

Breakfast

Coconut Fig Bars (p. 74)

YIELD: 12 servings
SERVING SIZE: 1 bar (2 by 2½-inches square)

- ½ cup coconut flour
- ½ cup old-fashioned rolled oats
- 1 cup unsweetened applesauce
- ¼ cup Date Honey (p. 212)
- 1 cup chopped dried figs
- 2 tablespoons chopped pecans
- 1 tablespoon flaxseed meal (optional)
- 1 tablespoon unsweetened shredded coconut
- ½ teaspoon cinnamon

Snickerdoodle Smoothie (p. 78)

YIELD: 2 servings
SERVING SIZE: about 1½ cups

- 6 ounces silken tofu
- ½ cup unsweetened almond or rice milk
- ¼ cup Date Honey (p. 212)
- 2 frozen bananas, peeled, sliced (about 2 cups)
- 1 teaspoon cinnamon
- ⅛ teaspoon nutmeg

Tropical Fruit Salad (p. 80)

YIELD: 6 servings
SERVING SIZE: about 1 cup

- 2 cups sliced strawberries
- 3 kiwifruit, peeled and quartered
- 1½ cups orange segments, cut into 1-inch pieces
- 1 cup red seedless grapes, halved
- 1 cup fresh pineapple chunks, diced

Appetizers and Snacks

Almond Butter Bites (p. 82)

YIELD: 6 – 8 servings
SERVING SIZE: 2 – 3 balls

- ½ cup almond butter
- ¼ cup raw sunflower seeds
- ¼ cup raisins
- ¼ cup chopped almonds
- 2 tablespoons unsweetened shredded coconut
- ¼ teaspoon cinnamon

Gimme More Granola (p. 89)

YIELD: 8 servings
SERVING SIZE: about ¼ cup

- ¼ cup chopped dried plums (prunes) or pitted dates
- ¼ cup water
- 1 cup old-fashioned rolled oats
- 2 tablespoons unsweetened apple juice
- 1 tablespoon extra-virgin olive oil

¼ cup raisins

2 tablespoons chopped almonds

2 tablespoons chopped walnuts

2 tablespoons raw sunflower seeds

2 tablespoons unsweetened shredded coconut

Salsa (p. 96)

YIELD: 12 servings

SERVING SIZE: about ¼ cup

3 – 4 large tomatoes, unpeeled, unseeded, quartered

1 (10-ounce) can diced tomatoes and green chilies, undrained

½ cup chopped green bell peppers

½ cup chopped red bell peppers

½ cup chopped red onion

1 serrano pepper, seeded and chopped

¼ cup packed fresh cilantro or parsley

2 – 3 cloves garlic, minced

1 tablespoon fresh lime juice

½ teaspoon salt

¼ teaspoon cumin

Spinach-Artichoke Dip (p. 97)

YIELD: 8 servings

SERVING SIZE: about ¼ cup

8 ounces firm tofu, drained

1 cup chopped canned artichokes, drained; reserve 2 tablespoons canned juices

½ (10-ounce) package frozen chopped spinach, thawed, squeezed dry

1 teaspoon dried basil

1 teaspoon salt

⅛ teaspoon pepper

2 teaspoons extra-virgin olive oil

¼ cup diced onion

2 cloves garlic, minced

Tortilla Chips (p. 100)

YIELD: 4 – 6 servings

SERVING SIZE: 8 – 12 chips

1 cup yellow cornmeal

½ cup warm water

½ tablespoon fresh lime juice

½ teaspoon salt

⅛ teaspoon pepper

Vegetables

Baked Potato Chips (p. 139)

YIELD: 4 servings

SERVING SIZE: about 1 cup

2 pounds russet baking potatoes, peeled

1 tablespoon extra-virgin olive oil

½ teaspoon salt

⅛ teaspoon pepper

Classic Tomato Sauce (p. 140)

YIELD: 8 servings

SERVING SIZE: about ½ cup

1 tablespoon extra-virgin olive oil

½ cup chopped onion

2 cloves garlic, minced

1 (29-ounce) can tomato puree

1 (6-ounce) can tomato paste

½ cup water

1 bay leaf

1 teaspoon dried basil

1 teaspoon dried parsley

½ teaspoon salt

⅛ teaspoon pepper

Marinated Zucchini (p. 150)

YIELD: 8 servings
SERVING SIZE: about ½ cup

- 2 pounds zucchini, unpeeled
- 1½ tablespoons olive oil
- 1 clove garlic, minced
- 1½ teaspoons dried oregano flakes
- ½ teaspoon salt
- ⅛ teaspoon pepper
- 1 teaspoon fresh lemon juice

Pan-Roasted Broccoli and Cauliflower (p. 152)

YIELD: 8 servings
SERVING SIZE: about 1 cup

- 1 tablespoon extra-virgin olive oil
- ½ cup diced onion
- 3 cups broccoli florets
- 3 cups cauliflower florets
- 1 tablespoon fresh oregano or 1 teaspoon dried oregano flakes
- ½ teaspoon salt

Salads, Soups, and Main Dishes

Butternut Squash and Broccoli Salad (p. 103)

YIELD: 4 servings
SERVING SIZE: about 1¼ cups

- 1½ pounds butternut squash, peeled and cut into 1-inch cubes (about 3 cups)
- 3 cups chopped broccoli florets, cut into 1-inch pieces
- ½ cup canned black beans, rinsed and drained

- 1½ tablespoons extra-virgin olive oil
- 2 tablespoons chopped fresh parsley
- ¼ teaspoon dried basil
- ¼ teaspoon garlic powder
- ⅛ teaspoon thyme
- 2 tablespoons toasted chopped walnuts for garnish
- 2 tablespoons toasted pumpkin seeds (pepitas) for garnish

Spinach Salad (p. 110)

YIELD: 4 servings
SERVING SIZE: about 1 cup

- 4 cups torn fresh spinach, loosely packed
- 1 cup canned chickpeas, rinsed and drained
- 1 cup chopped carrots
- 1 cup chopped sugar snap peas
- 1 cup chopped tomatoes, unpeeled, unseeded
- 1 cup chopped zucchini
- 2 tablespoons raw sunflower seeds

Rice, Bean, and Sweet Potato Soup (p. 128)

YIELD: 8 servings
SERVING SIZE: about 1¼ cups

- 8 cups water or Vegetable Broth (p. 212)
- 1 pound sweet potatoes (about 3 cups), peeled, diced
- 1 (15-ounce) can black beans, rinsed and drained
- 2 cups cooked brown rice
- ½ cup chopped celery
- ½ cup chopped onion
- 2 tablespoons chopped fresh parsley or 2 teaspoons dried parsley
- 1 bay leaf

1 teaspoon thyme

1 teaspoon salt

⅛ teaspoon pepper

Taco Soup (p. 130)

YIELD: 8 servings
SERVING SIZE: about 1 cup

1 tablespoon extra-virgin olive oil

½ cup diced onion

4 cups water or Vegetable Broth (p. 212)

1 (14.5 ounce) can diced tomatoes, undrained

1 (15-ounce) can black beans, rinsed and drained

1 (15-ounce) can pinto beans, rinsed, drained, and mashed

1 (15-ounce) can corn kernels, drained

2 cups cooked polenta or ½ cup dry polenta

1 tablespoon Taco Seasoning (p. 212)

1 teaspoon salt

⅛ teaspoon pepper
Tortilla Chips (p. 209)

Chipotle Black Bean Burgers (p. 163)

YIELD: 6 servings
SERVING SIZE: 1 burger

1 (15-ounce) can black beans, rinsed and drained

1 cup mashed cooked sweet potatoes (about 1 large sweet potato, peeled)

¼ cup oat flour (see Recipe Notes)

½ tablespoon dried parsley

¼ teaspoon chipotle chili pepper seasoning

¼ teaspoon garlic powder

¼ teaspoon salt

⅛ teaspoon pepper

Flatbread Pizza with Macadamia Nut Cheese (p. 166)

YIELD: 8 servings
SERVING SIZE: 1 slice

Pizza

2½ cups whole wheat flour

2 tablespoons flaxseed meal

1 teaspoon salt

1 cup warm water

1 cup Spinach-Artichoke Dip (p. 209)

1 cup Classic Tomato Sauce (p. 209)

Macadamia Nut Cheese

½ cup raw macadamia nuts

Toppings

Green peppers, mushrooms, black olives, onions, roasted red bell peppers

Lentil-Spinach "Meatballs" (p. 171)

YIELD: 8 servings
SERVING SIZE: 2 balls

½ cup dry lentils, sorted and rinsed

1½ cups Vegetable Broth (p. 212) or water

½ cup diced onion

1 clove garlic, minced

1½ teaspoons extra-virgin olive oil

1 cup finely chopped white button mushrooms

½ (10-ounce) package frozen chopped spinach, thawed, squeezed dry

½ cup oat flour (see Recipe Notes)

2 tablespoons finely chopped walnuts

2 tablespoons flaxseed meal

1 teaspoon dried basil

1 teaspoon dried parsley

½ teaspoon garlic powder

½ teaspoon salt

Other

Date Honey (p. 87)

YIELD: 12 servings
SERVING SIZE: about 1 tablespoon

- 1 cup pitted dates (about 6 – 8 Medjool or 18 – 20 Deglet Noor)
- 1 cup water
- ½ teaspoon cinnamon

Taco Seasoning (p. 98)

YIELD: 48 servings
SERVING SIZE: ¼ teaspoon

- 2 tablespoons chili powder
- 1 tablespoon cumin
- 1 teaspoon garlic powder
- 1 teaspoon paprika
- 1 teaspoon onion powder
- ½ teaspoon oregano
- ⅛ teaspoon cayenne pepper

Vegetable Broth (p. 134)

YIELD: 8 servings
SERVING SIZE: about 1 cup

- 8 cups water
- 1 onion, quartered
- 2 carrots, unpeeled and cut into 2-inch chunks
- 2 celery stalks, cut into 2-inch chunks, leafy tops included
- 1 russet potato, unpeeled and cut into 2-inch chunks
- 4 white button mushrooms, sliced
- ⅛ cup fresh parsley or ½ tablespoon dried parsley
- 2 cloves garlic, peeled
- 1 bay leaf
- 1 teaspoon dried thyme
- 1 teaspoon salt
- 6 peppercorns

Ingredients Lists for the Week 3 Suggested Meal Plan (p. 67)

Note: Page numbers next to recipe titles indicate the page on which you can find the complete recipe in part 3, "The Food." Page numbers within ingredients lists are for the page an ingredients list appears on in this appendix. No recipe variations are given in this section. Refer to the recipes in "The Food" for recipe variations.

Breakfast

Cinnamon Baked Apples (p. 73)

YIELD: 4 servings
SERVING SIZE: about ½ cup

- 2 cups thinly sliced apples, unpeeled (about 2 apples)
- 1 cup unsweetened apple juice
- ⅛ teaspoon cinnamon

Fall Harvest Oatmeal (p. 75)

YIELD: 2 servings
SERVING SIZE: about 1 cup

- ½ recipe Cinnamon Baked Apples (p. 213)
- ⅔ cup old-fashioned rolled oats
- 4 Medjool dates, pitted, chopped (about ¼ cup)
- 2 tablespoons chopped pecans
- ¼ cup apple juice (from Cinnamon Baked Apples recipe)

Fruit Pizza (p. 76)

YIELD: 6 – 8 servings
SERVING SIZE: 1 slice

Crust
- 1½ cups almond flour (meal)
- ½ cup roughly chopped pitted dates
- ½ cup chopped pecans
- ¼ cup unsweetened apple juice

Fruit Sauce
- ¼ cup Date Honey (p. 217)
- ½ cup sliced strawberries

Topping Ideas
Sliced apples, bananas, blueberries, grapes, kiwifruit, mangoes, oranges, peaches, pineapples, strawberries

Appetizers and Snacks

Corn Muffins (p. 86)

YIELD: 12 servings
SERVING SIZE: 2 mini muffins or 1 regular muffin

- 1½ cups yellow cornmeal
- ½ cup unsweetened almond or rice milk
- ¼ cup water
- 1 tablespoon Date Honey (p. 217) (optional)
- 1 tablespoon extra-virgin olive oil
- ¾ cup fresh or frozen corn kernels
- ¼ cup chopped green onions (green parts only)
- ½ teaspoon salt

Green Salsa Bean Dip (p. 90)

YIELD: 16 servings
SERVING SIZE: about 2 tablespoons

- 1 (15-ounce) can great northern beans, rinsed and drained
- 1 (10-ounce) can diced tomatoes and green chilies, undrained

2 cups chopped kale or spinach, lightly packed
2 cloves garlic, minced
½ teaspoon salt

Oatmeal Raisin Cookies (p. 93)

YIELD: 18–20 servings
SERVING SIZE: 1 cookie

1 cup old-fashioned rolled oats
1 cup almond flour or oat flour (see Recipe Notes)
1 cup creamy cashew butter, almond butter, or peanut butter
½ cup unsweetened applesauce
⅓ cup Date Honey (p. 217)
½ cup raisins
2 tablespoons chopped walnuts
1 teaspoon cinnamon

Pesto (p. 94)

YIELD: 6 servings
SERVING SIZE: about 2 tablespoons

2 tablespoons extra-virgin olive oil
3 cups fresh spinach leaves, packed
¼ cup chopped green onions
¼ cup pine nuts or walnuts
2 cloves garlic, minced
½ cup packed fresh basil leaves
¼ teaspoon salt

Petite Pecan Pies (p. 94)

YIELD: 4 servings
SERVING SIZE: 2 pies

8 Medjool dates
8 pecan halves

Vegetables

Ginger-Garlic Baby Carrots (p. 144)

YIELD: 6 servings
SERVING SIZE: about ½ cup

1 pound baby carrots or 1 pound carrots, peeled and cut into 2-inch pieces
½ tablespoon extra-virgin olive oil
2 tablespoons minced onion
1 clove garlic, minced
½ teaspoon minced fresh ginger root or ⅛ teaspoon dried ginger
⅛ teaspoon salt
Grated ginger root

Mashed Potato and Corn Casserole (p. 151)

YIELD: 12 servings
SERVING SIZE: about ½ cup

2 pounds russet potatoes, peeled and cubed
¼ cup unsweetened almond milk or soy milk
1 (14.5-ounce) can corn kernels, drained
2 tablespoons chopped fresh parsley
1 teaspoon salt
⅛ teaspoon pepper
½ tablespoon extra-virgin olive oil
½ cup diced onion
½ cup chopped green onion (green parts only)
2 cloves garlic, minced

Topping
¼ cup yellow cornmeal
½ tablespoon extra-virgin olive oil
½ teaspoon garlic powder

Green Beans with Toasted Walnuts (p. 146)

YIELD: 6 servings
SERVING SIZE: about ½ cup

- 1 pound fresh or frozen green beans
- ½ tablespoon extra-virgin olive oil
- ½ teaspoon salt
- ¼ teaspoon tarragon
- ⅛ teaspoon pepper
- 2 tablespoons finely diced toasted walnuts

Pesto Spaghetti Squash (p. 152)

YIELD: 6 servings
SERVING SIZE: about ½ cup

- 2 pounds spaghetti squash
- 1 recipe Pesto (p. 214)

Salads, Soups, and Main Dishes

Mediterranean Black Bean Salad (p. 105)

YIELD: 12 servings
SERVING SIZE: about ½ cup

- 2 (15-ounce) cans black beans, rinsed and drained
- 1 cup chopped green bell peppers
- 1 cup chopped red bell peppers
- 1 cup chopped tomatoes, unpeeled, unseeded
- 1 cup chopped avocados, cut into ½-inch cubes (about 1 medium avocado)
- ½ cup diced onion
- ¼ cup chopped fresh parsley or cilantro

Dressing

- 2 tablespoons fresh lime juice
- 1 tablespoon extra-virgin olive oil
- 2 cloves garlic, minced
- ½ teaspoon salt

Ozarks Sunset Fruit Salad (p. 107)

YIELD: 4 servings
SERVING SIZE: about 1¼ cups

- 2 cups torn fresh spinach leaves, packed, stems removed
- 2 cups torn romaine lettuce, packed
- 2 cups orange segments, cut into 1-inch pieces
- 2 kiwifruit, peeled and cut into half moons
- 1 cup sliced strawberries
- ½ cup blueberries
- ¼ cup sliced or slivered almonds, toasted

Jamaican Chili (p. 126)

YIELD: 4 servings
SERVING SIZE: about 1¼ cups

- 1 tablespoon extra-virgin olive oil
- 1 cup chopped onion
- 1½ cups chopped yellow bell pepper, seeded
- 2 cloves garlic, minced
- 1 cup water or Vegetable Broth (p. 217)
- 1 (15-ounce) can black beans, rinsed and drained
- 1 (15-ounce) can cannellini beans, rinsed and drained
- 1 (15-ounce) can kidney beans, rinsed and drained
- 1 (14.5-ounce) can diced tomatoes, undrained
- 1 teaspoon cumin
- 1 teaspoon paprika
- ½ teaspoon salt
- ¼ cup chopped fresh parsley

Vegetable Bean Soup (p. 133)

YIELD: 8 servings
SERVING SIZE: about 1¼ cups

- 1 tablespoon extra-virgin olive oil
- ½ cup chopped onion
- ½ cup chopped carrots
- ½ cup chopped celery
- 1 clove garlic, minced
- 6 cups water
- 1 (8-ounce) can tomato sauce
- 1 (14.5-ounce) can light red kidney beans, rinsed and drained
- 1 (15-ounce) can black-eyed peas, rinsed and drained
- 1 (14.5-ounce) can French-style green beans, drained
- 1 cup chopped yellow summer squash, unpeeled
- ½ tablespoon chili powder
- 1 bay leaf
- 1 teaspoon salt
- ⅛ teaspoon pepper
- 2 tablespoons chopped fresh parsley

Caribbean Wild Rice (p. 162)

YIELD: 6 servings
SERVING SIZE: about 1 cup

- 1 tablespoon extra-virgin olive oil
- ½ cup chopped onion
- 1 clove garlic, minced
- 1 (8-ounce) can unsweetened pineapple tidbits, juice reserved
- 2 tablespoons Bragg's Liquid Aminos or soy sauce
- 1½ tablespoons fresh lime juice
- 1 cup sliced carrots
- 1 cup chopped snow peas

- 1 cup chopped zucchini
- ½ cup chopped jarred roasted red bell peppers, drained
- ½ cup black beans, rinsed and drained
- ½ cup canned chickpeas, rinsed and drained
- 2 cups cooked wild rice
  Avocado slices
  Chopped macadamia nuts

Greek-Style Stuffed Peppers (p. 168)

YIELD: 6 servings
SERVING SIZE: about 2 pepper halves

- 1 tablespoon extra-virgin olive oil
- ½ cup chopped onion
- ½ cup diced zucchini
- 1 clove garlic, minced
- 1 (8-ounce) can tomato sauce
- 3 chopped canned artichokes, drained
- ½ cup chopped black olives
- 1 teaspoon dried oregano flakes or 1 tablespoon chopped fresh oregano
- 1 teaspoon dried parsley or 1 tablespoon chopped fresh parsley
- ½ teaspoon salt
- 6 medium bell peppers (green, orange, red, and/or yellow)
- 2 cups cooked quinoa
- 1½ tablespoons pine nuts

Spinach-Zucchini Casserole (p. 181)

YIELD: 6 servings
SERVING SIZE: about 1 cup

- 1 (28-ounce) can diced tomatoes, undrained
- 2 cloves garlic, minced
- ½ tablespoon dried basil
- ½ tablespoon dried oregano flakes
- ½ tablespoon dried parsley
- 1 teaspoon salt

1½ pounds zucchini, sliced into ½-inch rounds (about 2 – 3 medium zucchini)

3 cups packed fresh spinach, stems removed

1 cup thinly sliced onion, sliced pole to pole (see Recipe Notes)

Cooked brown rice, lentils, or quinoa

Other

Date Honey (p. 87)

YIELD: 12 servings
SERVING SIZE: about 1 tablespoon

1 cup pitted dates (about 6 – 8 Medjool or 18 – 20 Deglet Noor)

1 cup water

½ teaspoon cinnamon

Vegetable Broth (p. 134)

YIELD: 8 servings
SERVING SIZE: about 1 cup

8 cups water

1 onion, quartered

2 carrots, unpeeled and cut into 2-inch chunks

2 celery stalks, cut into 2-inch chunks, leafy tops included

1 russet potato, unpeeled and cut into 2-inch chunks

4 white button mushrooms, sliced

⅛ cup fresh parsley or ½ tablespoon dried parsley

2 cloves garlic, peeled

1 bay leaf

1 teaspoon dried thyme

1 teaspoon salt

6 peppercorns

Index of Recipes

Note: page numbers in boldface refer to the page the full recipe appears on. All other page numbers are to mentions of the recipe.

Share Your Thoughts

With the Author: Your comments will be forwarded to the author when you send them to *zauthor@zondervan.com*.

With Zondervan: Submit your review of this book by writing to *zreview@zondervan.com*.

Free Online Resources at
www.zondervan.com

Zondervan AuthorTracker: Be notified whenever your favorite authors publish new books, go on tour, or post an update about what's happening in their lives at www.zondervan.com/authortracker.

Daily Bible Verses and Devotions: Enrich your life with daily Bible verses or devotions that help you start every morning focused on God. Visit www.zondervan.com/newsletters.

Free Email Publications: Sign up for newsletters on Christian living, academic resources, church ministry, fiction, children's resources, and more. Visit www.zondervan.com/newsletters.

Zondervan Bible Search: Find and compare Bible passages in a variety of translations at www.zondervanbiblesearch.com.

Other Benefits: Register yourself to receive online benefits like coupons and special offers, or to participate in research.

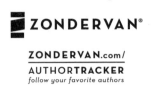

ZONDERVAN®

ZONDERVAN.com/
AUTHORTRACKER
follow your favorite authors